SportsVision

Training for Better Performance

Thomas A. Wilson

Jeff Falkel

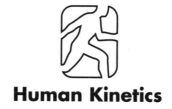

Human Kinetics

Library of Congress Cataloging-in-Publication Data

Wilson, Thomas A., 1961-
  SportsVision : training for better performance / Thomas A. Wilson,
Jeff Falkel.
      p. cm.
Includes bibliographical references and index.
  ISBN 0-7360-4569-4 (hard)
  1. Visual training. 2. Physical education and training. 3.
Sports--Physiological aspects. I. Title: Sports Vision. II. Falkel,
Jeff. III. Title.
  RE960.W53 2004
  617.7--dc22

                              2003015758

ISBN: 0-7360-4569-4

Acquisitions Editor: Michael S. Bahrke, PhD; **Developmental Editors:** Rebecca Crist, Renee Thomas Pyrtel; **Assistant Editors:** Sandria Washington, Sandra Merz Bott, Ann Augspurger; **Copyeditor:** Karen Bojda; **Proofreader:** Jim Burns; **Indexer:** Betty Frizzéll; **Permission Manager:** Dalene Reeder; **Graphic Designer:** Andrew Tietz; **Graphic Artist:** Angela K. Snyder; **Photo Manager:** Kareema McLendon; **Cover Designer:** Jack W. Davis; **Photographer (cover):** Grant Halverson, Getty Images; **Photographer (interior):** Andy Boudreau; **Art Manager:** Kelly Hendren; **Illustrator:** Kelly Hendren; **Printer:** United Graphics

Printed in the United States of America   10 9 8 7 6 5 4 3 2 1

Human Kinetics
Web site: www.HumanKinetics.com

United States: Human Kinetics
P.O. Box 5076
Champaign, IL 61825-5076
800-747-4457
e-mail: humank@hkusa.com

Canada: Human Kinetics
475 Devonshire Road Unit 100
Windsor, ON N8Y 2L5
800-465-7301 (in Canada only)
e-mail: orders@hkcanada.com

Europe: Human Kinetics
107 Bradford Road
Stanningley
Leeds LS28 6AT, United Kingdom
+44 (0) 113 255 5665
e-mail: hk@hkeurope.com

Australia: Human Kinetics
57A Price Avenue
Lower Mitcham, South Australia 5062
08 8277 1555
e-mail: liaw@hkaustralia.com

New Zealand: Human Kinetics
Division of Sports Distributors NZ Ltd.
P.O. Box 300 226 Albany
North Shore City
Auckland
0064 9 448 1207
e-mail: blairc@hknewz.com

To our families, who have given our work meaning, and to all the athletes and coaches we have had the privilege of working with, who have shown us the light of *SportsVision.*

CONTENTS

ICON KEY

These icons are used in chapters 4 and 5 as shorthand for different types of loading. Two types of loading, balance and motor skills, also have icons for specific exercises. You will see these icons in the exercises in chapter 4 and in the sport-specific programs in chapter 5.

B = **Balance**

 = Single foot balance   = 4-in-1 balance beam   = Teeter board

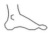 = Tennis balls   = Mini trampoline   = Balance ball

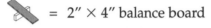 = 2" × 4" balance board

MS = **Motor Skills**

 = Abdominal exercises   = Backward running   = Jogging in place

= Jumping jacks   = Lunges   = Side-to-side running

 = Squats   = Running

RE = **Resistance Exercises**

 = with dumbbells   = in supine position

MET = **Metronome**   **GW** = **Gaze work**

J = **Juggling**   **HM** = **Head movements**

OEO = **One eye open**   **PLYO** = **Plyometrics**

SL = **Strobe light**   **RE** = **Resistance exercises**

PREFACE

This book is written for coaches, athletes, exercise physiologists, parents, and anyone else interested in enhancing the athlete's training experience and dramatically improving the athlete's success on the field or court. This book was conceived over 12 years ago, after an introductory lecture on sports vision to a group of physical therapy students. We perceived the need for a text written not for eye care professionals but rather for coaches who had a desire to improve their athletes' visual skills and thus their athletes' overall performance.

Training to enhance vision in sports is not a new concept. Sports vision training has been done primarily in laboratory or clinical environments, at significant cost to the athlete. In addition, most of the equipment used in the lab can be used only in clinical settings, not out on the field, where the athlete actually competes. This book is designed to allow any athlete, coach, or parent to perform simple yet effective sports vision training exercises with little expense, and most important, the athlete and coach can perform the exercises on the field or court, where exercise specificity results in the best long-term carryover to the visual system. This text brings sports vision training to any athlete, regardless of age or ability. Any athlete who works at *SportsVision* will see tremendous results.

One of the unique aspects of our concept of *SportsVision* is that training is a dynamic activity that should replicate the actual visual demands of the sport as closely as possible. Most other sports vision programs involve static, seated training of the visual system that just does not occur in the majority of sport skills or during competition.

Most parents cannot afford to send their young athletes to a sports vision clinic or laboratory. With this book, every person who wants to improve vision and actual sports performance can now afford to.

Why is the book needed now? At the time of publication, no other books address sports vision enhancement and training, with the exception of an outstanding book on sports vision specifically for golf by Dr. Craig Farnsworth. Therefore, we saw a compelling need to address vision in a sport-specific context for a wide variety of sports. Our book is unique among all previous sports vision books in that it is the only one that takes sports vision out of the lab and onto the field and addresses the specific needs of many particular sports.

For each of the sports addressed in the book, we evaluated the visual demands of the sport. For example, there is a need in baseball and hockey to track small, high-velocity projectiles. We examined the demands of gaze (where the eyes are looking while playing that sport). That is critical in racket sports and volleyball. We looked at speed of eye movements required by the sport, such as lacrosse and football. Finally, we integrated the coordination, balance, and visual needs of specific sports and designed appropriate *SportsVision* exercises to meet those demands as well.

We have addressed the visual needs and provided training exercises for 17 different sports. It would be impossible to address every single sport. However, most sports that are not specifically discussed here are similar to some sport that is discussed; therefore, a sports vision training program can be modified to meet the demands of that sport. Many exercises for each of the different components of *SportsVision* are presented, and modifications of these exercises for the specific demands of each sport are addressed.

We hope to receive a great deal of correspondence relating to the unique and fun *SportsVision* exercises we have provided in this book. With your help, we can incorporate adaptations into the next edition of our *SportsVision* book. Please feel free to send your suggestions or questions to

Dr. Jeff Falkel
VDP Enterprises
8415 S. Wildcat St.
Littleton, CO 80126-2019
E-mail: jfalkel@att.net

ACKNOWLEDGMENTS

This book would never have become a reality were it not for the efforts, encouragement, and support of many people. We would specifically like to thank Dr. Mike Bahrke, our acquisitions editor at Human Kinetics, who saw the potential and gave us his wholehearted support. We would also like to give our most sincere thanks to our developmental editors, Ms. Rebecca Crist and Ms. Renee Thomas Pyrtel, who are awesome and have really made this project look good. All the photos were graciously provided for us by our dear friend Mr. Andy Boudreau, and we are grateful for the diligence and time of our subjects Tim Falkel and Garrett Wilson. We would also like to acknowledge the developmental optometrists and their staffs who came up with the original concepts for some of the exercises in this book. Our thanks go out to the professionals who provided us with such detailed and pertinent reviews, Dr. Craig Farnsworth, Dr. Don Chu, Mr. Roger Earle, and Mr. Dan Wathan. Finally, our most sincere thanks go out to all the athletes and coaches around the country who have shown us how valuable *SportsVision* really is.

INTRODUCTION

When an athlete takes the field of play, many things go through his head. Where is the ball? Where are my teammates? Where are the opponents? What effect does the weather have on the game? Probably the last thing that enters an athlete's mind is, How is my visual system working at this particular moment in the game? Yet athletes should be completely in tune with vision in order to perform at their best. Every sport involves the visual system in one way or another, yet very few coaches or athletes spend any time training the visual system to perform optimally during competition. Some coaches might argue that wrestling or swimming does not involve the visual system. However, as you will find out, vision is not seeing alone. Wrestlers, swimmers, and athletes in other sports thought to be nonvisual typically need to be able to visualize to perform at their best. The wrestler needs to visualize the next move before he performs it. The swimmer needs to visualize their stroke mechanics to achieve optimal propulsion. By "seeing with the mind's eye," the athlete is able to visualize the skill about to be performed. Visualization can be taught, as can many other visual perceptual skills. To perform at the highest level of competition, athletes have to be in tune with their visual motor and visual perceptual systems. Most athletes would never think about going into a competition without having practiced their skills and improved their sport-specific strength and conditioning before the game. The same should hold true for *SportsVision* training exercises. These activities, like any other component of the athlete's training regime, are necessary for optimal preparation for competition.

Whenever we introduce *SportsVision* training to coaches who were formerly athletes, they universally respond that they wish that someone had told them about *SportsVision* when they were still competing. They are equally thankful that we have introduced it to them as coaches, giving them the opportunity to expose their players to these techniques. *SportsVision* training is rooted in exercise physiology, visual rehabilitation, and various aspects of kinesiology and biomechanics. *SportsVision* training allows athletes to improve their visual skills and thus their performance skills. The improvements from *SportsVision* training in eye movement skills, focusing skills, peripheral visual awareness, and visual perceptual skills will carry over to the field of play, helping athletes perform their best and helping them reach the next level, no matter what level they are currently competing at. *SportsVision* gives even elite athletes an important edge over the competition. From youth leagues to professionals, any athlete's visual skills can be improved to enhance sport performance. We hope that this book helps coaches and athletes at all levels and in all sports appreciate the value of a superior visual system.

These days, performance-enhancing products are everywhere in the sports market. Controversies and scandals about the use of steroids and other performance-enhancing supplements abound. Some athletes in every sport are tempted to use performance-enhancing supplements or products, no matter what the cost or the long-term consequences. Coaches at all levels of sport routinely are asked about the use of performance-enhancement products. We have been asked by parents of youth swimmers, soccer players, and baseball players as young as 10 years old if we thought their children would benefit from creatine, steroids, human growth hormone, and androstenedione. Rather than asking about sport drinks or how much pizza is too much, these parents are looking for a training edge for their children in the black hole of pharmaceutical intervention. Scientific knowledge is lacking about the long-term side effects for young athletes who use many performance-enhancing supplements and products that are available today.

In contrast, *SportsVision* training is a method of performance enhancement that has been proven to take athletes at all levels of competition to the next level, is totally safe and completely legal, and has only positive consequences both on and off the field. The first rule in medicine should also be the first rule in coaching: Do no harm. *SportsVision* is a tool that coaches can use in their athletes' training regime that is safe and effective.

There is a huge psychological aspect to performance enhancement, as demonstrated by the use of placebos such as "special jelly-beans" or the infamous "can of whoop-ass" that coaches use to fire up their teams. If an athlete thinks that a particular supplement or activity will make her faster or better able to beat the competition, it probably will work. We have shown that *SportsVision* training not only improves eye movement efficiency but also elicits an advantageous psychological response. In addition, clear, distinct, measurable, and proven physiological advantages that can enhance athletic performance are elicited by *SportsVision* training.

We hope this book shows coaches and athletes alike the value and benefit of *SportsVision* training to improve sport performance. We invite you to see how much better you can compete after adding *SportsVision* to your training regimen. Join us for the next millennium of sport training through *SportsVision*.

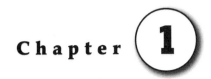

Chapter 1

What Is SportsVision?

Most coaches think that if their athletes can see 20/20, nothing more is needed in the visual arena. This misconception is common in youth sports and continues in professional sports as well. Studies have shown that even some elite Olympic athletes have not undergone a basic visual screening, and very few are exposed to any sort of training to enhance sports vision. The visual system is like any other motor system in the body. It can be trained and improved by sports vision exercises, just as athletes use sport-specific drills to improve overall performance.

The visual system responds to overload and progressive increases in the demands that the athlete places on it, just as the rest of the musculoskeletal system responds to the demands and overloads it faces in training. The perceptual component of the visual system can also be enhanced by *SportsVision* training. Visual perceptual training improves target areas such as visual memory, figure–ground perception, and laterality/directionality and helps the athlete better understand these concepts as they apply to a particular sport. The visual system has direct connections to the proprioceptive centers of the brain. These centers control awareness of the body's position in space, which is especially important during exercise and sport. Twenty percent of the fibers of the optic nerve go directly to the brain centers that regulate and control balance. This connection between the visual system and balance can quickly be demonstrated by trying to balance on one foot while your eyes are closed. By integrating visual perceptual and proprioceptive skills, the athlete develops the ability to focus directly on the task at hand and not be distracted by irrelevant parts of the game environment, such as surrounding opponents, the fans in the stands, or the color of the sky. It is no more correct to assume that all athletes have the same visual perceptual and visual motor skills than it is to assume that all athletes have the same natural athletic abilities. And just as many aspects of an athlete's abilities can be greatly enhanced by sport-specific skill training, the athlete's visual perceptual and visual motor abilities can be dramatically improved by *SportsVision* training. By using sport-specific vision enhancement activities in the training room, the weight room, and the field of play, coaches and athletes will see remarkable improvements in overall athletic performance. In addition, vision enhancement activities are fun and unique.

The basic premise of *SportsVision* is that stressing or loading the visual perceptual, visual motor, and visual proprioceptive systems during sport-specific training can better prepare the athlete for competition. Normally, an athlete encounters the most stress during the actual game or competition. Part of exercise and sport training is to overload the body's systems so as to prepare it to meet the demands of actual competition. Over the past several years, coaches in all sports have come to recognize the value of resistance training to improve the overall performance of their athletes. Even elite golfers have had dramatic improvements in performance as the result of sport-specific strength and conditioning programs. Without sufficient strength, endurance, and power, the demands of sport can be overwhelming and cause physical and mental exhaustion.

The same principles apply to *SportsVision* training. By overloading the visual system during sport-specific training, the athlete learns how to deal with visual and physical stress and is better able to overcome fatigue and breakdown caused by those stressors. Thus, in actual competition, athletes can perform at a higher level because they can deal with the visual and physical input with greater efficiency. How many times have you heard a sports announcer say, "He has great field awareness," "She has great vision," or "He has an uncanny ability to read the play"? Have you ever noticed that a particular athlete always seems to know where the ball is, where her teammates are, and where the opponents are? Studies have shown that such elite athletes possess not only great athletic skills but also great visual skills.

Another improvement in the overall conditioning and training of athletes is year-round training for sport. In the past, athletes would show up at training camp out of shape and would need time to become fit enough to play once the season started. Not anymore. Athletes are expected to show up at preseason training camps already in shape so that this preparation time can be better spent on skill and tactical development rather than conditioning activities. The athlete who shows up to camp visually fit will be that much better prepared for the rigors of the upcoming season. The purpose of *SportsVision* training is to give the athlete that extra edge needed to outplay and outperform less visually fit athletes. It is our hope that *SportsVision* training will soon be as much a part of the overall conditioning of an athlete as resistance training is today.

SportsVision training should be an adjunct to the overall conditioning and training of the athlete. By including *SportsVision* training in each training session, coaches will find that their athletes can perform better because they can better see what they should have been seeing all along. Today, in the fiercely competitive world of sports, too many coaches and athletes are tempted to resort to illegal means to gain an advantage over their opponents. It makes more sense to incorporate *SportsVision* into the overall training program to safely and legally help athletes achieve ultimate performance. The exercise programs outlined in this book can be incorporated into any form or level of sports training and serve to improve an athlete's performance not only on the field but in the classroom as well. Enhancing the coordination of the eyes improves reading speed and efficiency.

Elite athletes often refer to a peak performance as "being in the zone." For example, a basketball player who is "in the zone" and hits his first three-point attempt early in the game may have the confidence to shoot and make multiple three-point shots for the rest of the contest. After completing a *SportsVision* training program, many basketball players report that the rim seems to be larger and that they can visualize the arc of the shot with greater accuracy. Golfers can read the break of the green more accurately and consistently. Baseball and tennis players report that after *SportsVision* training the ball seems to move in slow motion as they prepare to hit or catch it, allowing them more time to set up and make a better play. The eyes lead the body. After training the visual system, it is much easier for an athlete to get in the zone because the visual system guides the motor system. A well-conditioned visual system more efficiently leads a well-tuned motor system to perform at its peak, time and time again.

Static Versus Dynamic Visual Acuity

Sight, or visual acuity, is the ability to see at a certain level of detail. To measure sight using the Snellen acuity scale, a person reads a row of letters or numbers from an eye chart a fixed distance away (appendix I.1). The chart is placed on a well-lit wall at approximately eye level, and the person should stand 20 feet away from the chart. He should cover his left eye first and read each line that can be seen clearly with the right eye. Repeat with the left eye.

Based on the distance and the size of the letter that the person can read accurately, a ratio is calculated that compares the person's ability to see with a normative standard. This standard ratio is commonly referred to as 20/20. If a person can see 20/20, she is considered to have normal sight. Many people can see 20/15, which is considered better than 20/20 because it means they can see letters at 20 feet that a person with standard sight can see at 15 feet. However, if a person's sight is classified as 20/100, this means that the person sees at 20 feet what a person with normal sight can see at 100 feet. A person with 20/100 sight needs some form of corrective lenses to see more normally. The best that a human can possibly see is theorized to be 20/07. (This level of sight, which is extremely rare, may soon be commonplace with advances in refractive laser surgery, which we discuss in more depth later in the book.) Visual acuity of 20/20 is considered to be good static visual acuity. Not every athlete needs both eyes or even one eye to have 20/20 sight. Many elite athletes have reduced acuity in one or both eyes and yet still perform at the elite level. This goes to show that visual acuity, or "seeing," is just one part of the visual puzzle. However, the rule of thumb is that every athlete's sight should be corrected to the best possible static visual acuity. Just as all athletes need a physical exam before every season, they should also have a complete eye exam before reporting to training camp.

Dynamic visual acuity is just as important to the athlete as static visual acuity. There are very few times in sport where nothing is moving. Therefore, it is extremely

External Devices to Correct Vision

For the athlete who needs some form of visual correction, it is our opinion that soft contact lenses are a far superior vision correction modality compared with traditional glasses or gas-permeable contact lenses. Soft contact lenses are safer because they will not shatter and allow greater peripheral awareness. Most prescriptions are available as disposable soft contact lenses, which allow the athlete to keep a backup set of lenses in a sports bag. Soft contact lenses are also very affordable.

However, contact lenses do not provide any protection from injury, as would be provided by polycarbonate spectacle lenses. If glasses are the only option, then sport goggles with polycarbonate lenses are a necessity. Polycarbonate lenses are shatterproof and provide 100 percent ultraviolet protection. Unfortunately, sport goggles do not fit easily inside some helmets; in addition, the athlete may be hesitant to wear sport goggles because of social stigma. A blow to the face can be very painful with sport goggles on. However, in sports such as handball, racquetball, and squash, where there is a significant risk of getting hit in the eye with either the ball or the racket, sport goggles are highly recommended for all athletes, even if they do not need visual correction.

important for athletes to be able to see as well as possible dynamically while engaged in their sports. Even an athlete with a static acuity of 20/10 cannot perform optimally without good dynamic acuity. *SportsVision* training for dynamic acuity can help any athlete have better vision on the field or court. Most athletes have never undergone a dynamic visual acuity test. There are many ways to administer a dynamic visual acuity test. However, the most common is the Landolt C test.

The C is a 20/40 letter size and is rotated at or above 100 revolutions per minute. The rotation is gradually slowed down until the athlete can correctly and consistently identify the position of the opening of the C as either up, down, left, or right. Several studies have shown that elite athletes can correctly identify the open position of the C at much higher revolution rates than can nonathletes. Static visual acuity can be corrected but not trained. Dynamic visual acuity can be trained. Various training activities for dynamic visual acuity are given throughout this book.

Basic Anatomy and Physiology of the Eye

The eye is a wonder of nature. Each eye has six extraocular muscles that attach the eye to the orbit, or eye socket, in the skull. These muscles can work individually or in combination to produce all the different movements of the eyes. Sometimes these muscles work in synergy with one another, and sometimes they work in opposition to produce a specific eye movement. For example, when the eyes look up and to the right, the superior rectus and inferior oblique muscles of both eyes, the lateral rectus muscle of the right eye, and the medial rectus muscle of the left eye contract simultaneously to achieve this simple movement. When our eyes cross, the medial rectus muscles of both eyes contract simultaneously. This is an example of an oppositional muscle action.

The six extraocular muscles of the eye, shown in figure 1.1, are similar to other skeletal muscles. They are striated muscles, and, like other skeletal muscles, which adapt to the stresses and demands that are placed on them, they adapt to exercise training. However, *SportsVision* training is not intended to strengthen these muscles, as they are already as strong as they need to be. *SportsVision* training is designed to improve the speed, coordination, and endurance of the extraocular muscles. Because the extraocular muscles of the eye are volitional muscles, similar to skeletal muscles, they can be controlled and trained with *SportsVision* exercises to perform at a higher level.

Here is a quick demonstration of how the speed of eye movement varies based on the number of muscles that are used to perform the task. While sitting in a chair, hold your thumbs up at eye level, approximately 16 inches away from your face, and 24 inches apart (see figure 1.2). Have a partner count the number of times your eyes can move back and forth from one thumb to the other in 60 seconds. Now, while keeping your head straight, stand and raise your arms so that your thumbs are approximately 12 inches above your nose but still 24 inches apart. Looking at

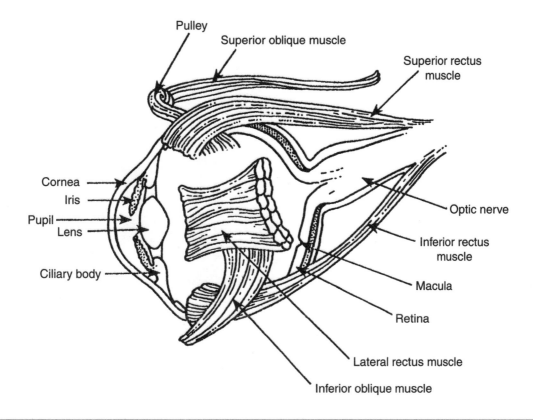

Pulley

Superior oblique muscle

Superior rectus muscle

Cornea

Iris

Pupil

Lens

Ciliary body

Optic nerve

Inferior rectus muscle

Macula

Retina

Lateral rectus muscle

Inferior oblique muscle

Figure 1.1 Five of the six extraocular muscles of the eye. The medial rectus muscle is on the opposite (inner) side of the eye and cannot be seen in this view.

them now requires what is called a superior gaze. Repeat the exercise. You should notice several changes. Most people report a decreased number of eye movements per minute when performing the exercise in the position of superior gaze. In addition, most people report a significant increase in fatigue for eye movements in superior gaze. Both of these changes are due to the additional number of muscles that are required to do the same activity in a different gaze position. *SportsVision* training can increase the speed, accuracy, and endurance of eye muscles in all positions of gaze.

There are nine cardinal positions of gaze: (1) up and left, or superior left; (2) up, or superior; (3) up and right, or superior right; (4) left; (5) straight ahead; (6) right; (7) down and left, or inferior left; (8) down, or inferior; and (9) down and right, or inferior right (see figure 1.3). In gaze exercises, left and right always refer to the athlete's left and right. In each gaze, multiple muscles work together to accomplish a particular eye movement. Some muscles must actively contract while the contralateral muscles need to relax. This is why coordination of the activity of the extraocular muscles is so critical for effective and accurate eye movements. One of the major benefits of *SportsVision* training is improving coordination of the extraocular muscles during athletic activities. Speed and accuracy of eye movements in superior gaze can benefit baseball, basketball, and volleyball players. By training these muscles to move faster and to fixate or judge the position of the ball more accurately as it moves in space, the athlete can react more rapidly and precisely to be in the best position to make the play.

Figure 1.2 *(a)* Sitting eye movement test. While sitting in a chair, hold your thumbs at eye level, approximately 16 inches away from your face, and 24 inches apart. Have a partner count the number of times your eyes can move back and forth from one thumb to the other in 60 seconds. *(b)* Standing eye movement test. Now, stand and raise your arms so that your thumbs are approximately 12 inches above your nose and still 24 inches apart, requiring a superior gaze to look at them. Repeat the test for 60 seconds. Record the differences between straight-ahead gaze and superior gaze. Because most athletes are standing, or at least in an upright posture during their sport, *SportsVision* tests and training should optimally be performed in the most sport-specific position.

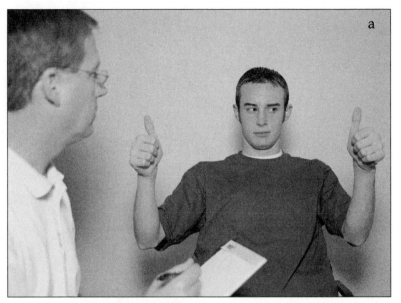

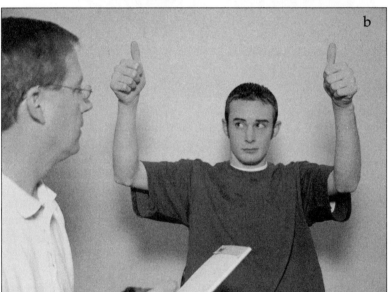

There are three other muscles in the eye. The first is the ciliary muscle. This muscle controls focusing, or accommodation. A frequent malady among athletes is accommodative insufficiency, or focusing insufficiency. This is a very easy problem to treat in athletes younger than 40 years of age. A temporary spasm of this muscle can cause blurriness, especially in activities that require quick near-to-far or far-to-near focusing. Many sports require the ability to refocus quickly from a nearby point to a point in the distance, or vice versa. This is called near–far focusing. If an athlete has an accommodative spasm, his ability to perform near–far activities can suffer greatly. *SportsVision* training can teach the athlete to relax the ciliary muscle and to refocus quickly and effectively from one distance to another.

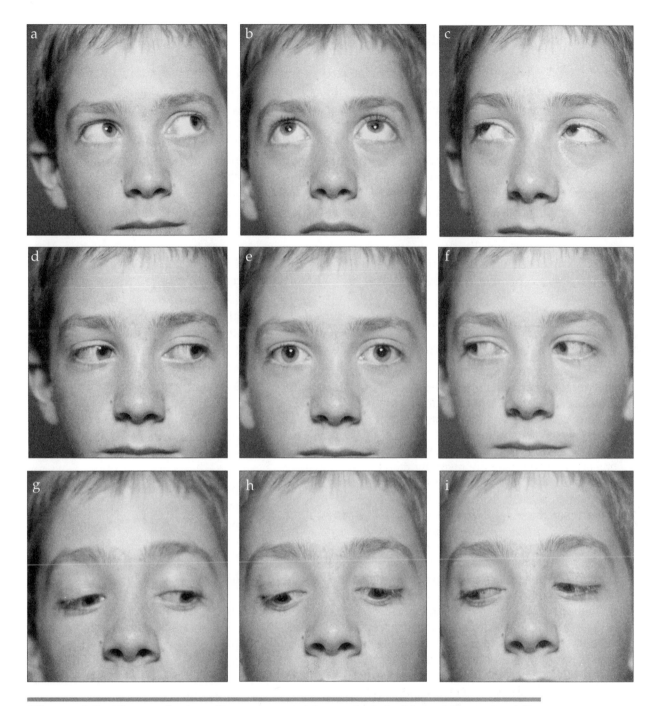

Figure 1.3 Nine cardinal positions of gaze: *(a)* superior left, *(b)* up, *(c)* superior right, *(d)* left, *(e)* straight ahead, *(f)* right, *(g)* inferior left, *(h)* down, and *(i)* inferior right.

The last two muscles in the eye are the sphincter and dilator muscles in the iris. These two muscles open and close the pupil to allow more or less light into the eye. Under various lighting conditions, such as bright sunlight, cloudy skies, or artificial light in a gym or arena, pupil size must vary to allow maximal contrast. The sphincter and dilator muscles are not voluntary and therefore cannot be trained with *SportsVision.* With age, these muscles are slower to react, and older athletes frequently require special tinted lenses to perform at their highest level.

Visual Motor Skills

Vision involves two basic categories of function: visual motor and visual perceptual skill. Visual motor skill is probably the easiest category to relate to sport-specific performance. If athletes cannot move their eyes quickly and effectively, they cannot perform sport-specific tasks optimally. In fact, one of the primary differences between good and elite-level athletes, other physical skills being equal, is that elite athletes can move their eyes more effectively and efficiently for the duration of the game. There are three basic ocular motor skills used in the visual motor system. They are vergence, focusing, and tracking. Consider the ocular motor skills needed to read this book. First, both eyes have to converge, that is, their views must cross, to see each word. Next, the eyes have to focus equally to make the words on the page clear. Finally, the eyes have to track from word to word to understand the text. Now consider the similar sequence out on the field of play. It is important for the eyes to be able to converge (or cross) as the ball comes toward the athlete or diverge (or uncross) as it goes away. It is also necessary for the athlete to be able to focus on the target and then track that target smoothly through space. We sometimes take these skills for granted in sports.

Tracking is the ability of the eyes to follow an object from one point to another. Tracking is done with two separate categories of eye movement. The first is pursuit eye movement, which is the ability of the eyes to smoothly follow an object through space, as when a wide receiver follows the ball from the release by the quarterback into his hands. The second category is saccadic eye movement, which is the quick jump of the eyes from one point to another. The wide receiver, after making the catch, uses saccadic eye movements to see who is going to try to tackle him. Pursuits and saccades are often used in sports and everyday life to perform both simple and complex tasks. Although many people take these eye movements for granted, these movements can be easily improved through training to enhance sport performance. For example, this chart can be used in a saccadic eye movement exercise:

LASIK Laser Vision Correction

Laser vision correction provides eye care practitioners, coaches, athletes, and athletic trainers with a huge conundrum: Laser vision correction can potentially provide an athlete with 20/20 vision. Laser in situ keratomileusis (LASIK) is the surgical method of choice at this time. A new surgical technology called wavefront technology, which has just recently been approved by the FDA, may actually provide optimal visual acuity. In the LASIK procedure, the eye is pressurized to six times its normal pressure. A blade called a keratome makes an incision across the cornea, thus creating a flap. The laser then molds the cornea so that the eye no longer needs external correction for 20/20 vision. The flap is then placed back onto the cornea, and the procedure is complete. The entire surgery lasts approximately five minutes, and by the next day, the athlete can return to normal activities, except for using eye makeup, submersion of the eye in chlorinated water, and contact sports. However, caution should be used in the immediate hours to weeks after the surgery, especially in contact sports.

The advantage of the LASIK procedure is that the athlete no longer needs glasses or contact lenses to see clearly. However, this procedure is recommended only for athletes over the age of 18 because younger athletes' prescriptions often change from year to year. Once the athlete's prescription has remained stable for one to two years and the athlete is over the age of 18, refractive laser surgery is presumed safe.

The corneal flap required in LASIK surgery seems to be stable in almost all instances. But many athletes experience extreme visual trauma on the field from a variety of foreign objects, and it has not been determined whether the corneal flap can withstand such extreme duress without dislodging.

W	I
K	T
C	P
A	N
V	B
H	R
E	Z

Hold this chart 12 inches away from your nose, and hold your head still. Start at the top of the chart, look at the letters from left to right row by row as quickly as possible, and see how long it takes your eyes to jump from letter to letter. Have a partner time you if you have difficulty timing yourself. Next, repeat the exercise while moving the book in a figure 8 pattern with the chart still 12 inches from your nose. See how much longer it takes to have your eyes jump from letter to letter. Repeat the figure 8 activity five times, and then redo the first version with the book stationary. Most people perform the stationary activity faster the second time, after having "loaded" the visual system by adding the pursuit eye movement task (i.e., the figure 8) to the stationary saccadic eye movement task. Research has proven that these visual motor skills can be improved through training to allow optimal visual motor performance during sports. The visual system actually performs better after it has been loaded, or stressed. We discuss loading the visual system with *SportsVision* training exercises in more detail in chapter 3.

The goal of *SportsVision* training is improving ocular motor skills to enhance not only visual performance but also sport performance. When you improve the ocular motor skills—vergence, focusing, and tracking—you improve athletic performance. Most coaches mistakenly assume that all eye movements are equally smooth in all their athletes. But assuming that every player has equal ocular motor skills is like assuming that every player can run the same speed or jump the same height. A person who has an overactive medial rectus in one eye, for example, can develop an inward turn of that eye, a condition known as esotropia, or lazy eye. A person with esotropia usually does not have the normal eye movement skills of a person without this condition. Unless there is a pathologic reason for a muscle disorder, *SportsVision* training can improve sport performance by helping athletes to visually track better while competing.

Coaches can perform this simple test of their athletes' visual motor skills. The athlete stands approximately two feet in front of the coach. The coach holds a pencil and instructs the athlete to follow the tip of the pencil while the coach moves it in various directions. The coach moves the pencil clockwise in a circle about two feet in diameter three times. Then the coach moves the pencil in a counterclockwise circle three times. Next, the coach moves the pencil in a horizontal figure 8 pattern for three repetitions. Repeat these three tasks while giving the athlete age-appropriate spelling or math problems to solve. The coach should note the athlete's eye movement patterns.

Virtually no two athletes will demonstrate equal tracking skills. Athletes with good tracking skills have smooth eye movements under all the test conditions. Athletes who have poor tracking skills have jerky movements, hesitate, or overshoot the target. In addition, many athletes' tracking abilities deteriorate significantly when cognitive activities are added. Better athletes are likely to have better tracking skills. But even the poorest trackers can be trained to have eye movement skills equal to the best tracker. We performed a similar tracking test on an NCAA Division I baseball team. About one in eight of the players had extremely poor tracking skills. When we asked which positions those poor trackers played, we discovered that, to a man, the poorest trackers on the team were pitchers. This is not to imply that college pitchers do not need superior visual skills; however, NCAA Division I pitchers do not have to bat. And because batting is a skill that requires tremendous tracking ability, it makes sense that the players who do not bat, and thus do not regularly practice tracking, have the poorest tracking skills.

Visual Perceptual Skills

Another important aspect of the visual system is the visual perceptual process. Visual perceptual skills include visual memory, which is the ability to see something, such as a play or diagram, and then remember what was seen; visualization, which is the ability to see something in the mind's eye; and figure–ground perception, which is the ability to recognize the significant part of what is seen, such as action on the field or court. Athletes need to be able to concentrate on the ball, the position of their teammates, and where an opponent is playing while ignoring the many distractions that occur during a sporting event. For example, a shortstop needs to have an uncanny ability to remain focused on catching the ball, looking to see where the runners are, and being aware of where the second baseman is in relation to the bag. Because she has practiced a particular play over and over again in practice, the shortstop can focus on actually making the catch, without deliberately looking at all the extraneous activities going on around her during the game.

Skiers can often be seen visualizing the course before a race. Once we asked a member of the University of Colorado ski team what he was visualizing before he started his race. He said, "I close my eyes, put my hand in front of my face, and go back and forth, because Coach wants us to do this! In reality, I have no idea what the course looks like in my head, but I don't want Coach to know that." After a brief lesson in visualization, this same skier told us after the next race that for the first time he was able to see the course in his head and that it made a world of difference in how he approached each successive combination of gates. *SportsVision* really does work!

Another important aspect of vision is the interaction between visual motor and visual perceptual skills. Magic Johnson, John Stockton, and Jason Kidd can miraculously make "no-look" passes; no one can figure out how they know a teammate will be in that exact place on the court at that precise moment in time. Olympic ski racers often somehow maintain their balance and stay on course despite what surely should have been a catastrophic fall. How many times has Tiger Woods "willed" the ball around a tree to get it onto the green, even though he could not see the green from where the ball was lying? These are all examples of athletes who have both highly developed motor skills and well-integrated visual motor and perceptual skills.

Eye–Hand and Eye–Foot Coordination

Two other basic skills that are often trained but rarely recognized as being components of sports vision are eye–hand and eye–foot coordination. By simply participating in a sport, athletes naturally tend to improve sport-specific skills, or they will stop playing that particular sport. Some athletes seem to have a natural gift for eye–hand or eye–foot coordination. For example, Michael Jordan and Pelé may never have done *SportsVision* training, but they both possess incredibly advanced eye–hand and eye–foot coordination in their respective sports. Some people think that this coordination has made the difference between their being great and their being the greatest in their sports. Improving eye–hand and eye–foot coordination through *SportsVision* will have a profound impact on skill, performance, and fun in sports. *Sports-Vision* takes a unique approach toward eye–foot coordination in sports that are traditionally considered eye–hand activities, such as basketball, volleyball, and baseball. While excellent coordination between eyes and hands is critical for these sports, athletes must also have outstanding eye–foot coordination to get into the best position to use their eye–hand coordination. Eye–foot coordination includes balance and agility. Plyometric exercises, such as jumping in place, standing jumps, multiple jumps, and bounding, are prime examples of eye–foot coordination activities that can be incorporated into a *SportsVision* training program for almost any athlete.

Ski Goggles and Sunglasses

Skiers and snowboarders *must* wear some form of ultraviolet (UV) eye protection while on the slopes. Ski goggles are a much safer form of eye protection during these sports than sunglasses for several reasons. Ski goggles provide complete protection from the sun, wind, snow, and UV light. Natural tearing that occurs while wearing sunglasses, but not ski goggles, decreases visual acuity. Ski goggles can be used easily with contact lenses, and some fit over prescription glasses. Many companies offer a prescription insert that fits inside the goggle and eliminates the need for contacts or eyeglasses while skiing.

Ski goggles come in a wide variety of tints and antireflective coatings. We have conducted several studies and found that a dark amber tint universally provides the best contrast on the slopes. This improves the athlete's ability to distinguish subtle changes on the snow surface. In fact, an athlete on the University of Colorado alpine ski team dramatically improved his performance by simply changing the tint of his ski goggles. With his old goggles, he was unable to clearly distinguish the red from the blue gates, and he therefore had to rely more on the tracks in the snow from the previous racers than his own view of the course. After changing his goggle tint to dark amber, he could clearly see each gate and dramatically improved his racing results. Richard Rokos, his coach and our good friend, told us, "He skis like God!" as a result of this subtle change in sports vision. The best tint is a very individual choice and the athlete should compare many tints under varied conditions.

Sunglasses may be a personal preference. While they may be helpful for contrast enhancement, the choice depends on the sport and the individual. Sunglasses can be beneficial in noncontact sports to improve contrast and provide UV protection while competing in the sunlight for prolonged periods. Many manufacturers offer tints to enhance contrast for a specific need; for example, a tennis player may benefit from a blue filter, while a trap shooter may benefit from a yellow filter. Again, each athlete should test samples of various tints in the playing arena to see which tint best meets his or her own requirements for contrast and glare elimination. Dr. John Peroff, an optometrist in Canada, suggests that skiers use the same tint in their sunglasses as in their ski goggles so that they require less time to adapt to the sunlight when they first start skiing.

Peripheral Awareness

The last area of vision we explore is peripheral awareness. Many eye care practitioners argue that peripheral vision is the same as peripheral awareness. We do not believe that this is true. Peripheral vision cannot be trained. Peripheral vision involves the ability of the rods and cones in the retina to detect light. There are approximately 100 million rods and 6 million cones in each eye at birth, and these numbers can only decrease with disease and aging. Because of this anatomic fact, peripheral vision cannot be changed by *SportsVision* training. However, *SportsVision* training can dramatically improve athletes' peripheral awareness, which means that they can readily identify objects in their peripheral vision more accurately and more quickly, so they do not have to use their central vision and expend unneeded energy to locate the opposition during a game. Peripheral awareness training is a very dynamic and necessary part of *SportsVision* training of athletes in almost every sport.

Body Alarm Reaction and *SportsVision*

It is common at all levels of competition for an athlete who normally performs without a flaw or difficulty most days to seem to simply fall apart during a particular game. What causes this dramatic change in performance? Part of this decrement in performance may be a consequence of the body alarm reaction, or BAR. Dr. Edward Godnig, an optometrist from Concord, New Hampshire, thinks that the BAR is the body's response to "an unexpected and sudden change in the environment" (Godnig 2001). Sympathetic overload exaggerates the body's natural fight or flight response. When an athlete is on the field or court, this fight or flight response is frequently evoked. Dr. Godnig illustrates this phenomenon using the example of a wide receiver in football. The fight or flight response takes place in an instant. As the ball is coming to the wide receiver, he needs to focus on the ball, watching it all the way into his hands and then catching it. At the same time, he is aware that the defender is probably getting ready to tackle him. The receiver also has the background distractions of the noise of the fans and the colors in the stadium while he is trying to see and catch the football. He must also be aware of where he is on the field and how many yards he needs for a first down or touchdown. Given all these demands on and distractions from his focus, an athlete with a heightened BAR is likely to drop even a ball that hits him right in the numbers. In contrast, an athlete who has a low BAR is able to focus clearly on the target and perform the task successfully. *SportsVision* training creates a visual overload in the athlete's normal training sessions that can reduce the athlete's BAR by allowing the athlete to focus on the most important object (i.e., the ball) and to block out extraneous distractions.

Sports Vision Testing and Evaluation

It is imperative that every athlete over the age of five receive a basic eye exam. This basic eye exam should include testing of near and far static visual acuity, color and depth perception, and basic refraction (evaluation of the need for prescription correction). After the age of 10, intraocular pressures should be evaluated. Intraocular pressure is the pressure of the fluid inside the eye. If the intraocular pressure becomes too high, it can lead to glaucoma, which destroys peripheral vision. In addition to a basic eye examination, sports vision testing includes detailed evaluations of visual motor skills, visual perceptual skills, eye–hand and eye–foot coordination, and peripheral awareness.

Why do sports vision testing? Sports vision testing gives insight into the player's ability to perform visually. Just as there are many more components to athletic strength and ability than just the one-repetition maximum (1RM), so too there are many more aspects to vision during sport than just static acuity. Sports vision testing provides a total picture of an athlete's visual motor and visual perceptual abilities. Sports vision testing also provides insight into the areas that need improvement or enhancement to help the athlete perform optimally. In chapter 3, we provide a *SportsVision* evaluation that can be performed with minimal equipment and yields valuable insight into the athlete's visual skills and abilities.

Who Benefits From *SportsVision* Training?

While all athletes can benefit from *SportsVision* training, every coach knows of athletes who just seem to misjudge the ball or get to where they need to be just half a second too late. These athletes can benefit the most from aggressive *SportsVision* training. Talented athletes who do not live up to their potential are also prime candidates for *SportsVision* training. But *SportsVision* training is easily implemented and is an extremely beneficial addition to all athletic programs for athletes of all ages and abilities. This book is designed to give the coaches, athletes, and parents the ability to structure a *SportsVision* program to assess and enhance the athlete's visual abilities.

Chapter ②

Basics of
SportsVision

One of the advantages of *SportsVision* training is that it can be modified to fit a variety of circumstances and settings, from a highly specialized clinical laboratory to a bare room (see figures 2.1 through 2.4). On the luxurious side, there are specialized sports vision clinics and laboratories in most cities around the country. These clinics use complex (and expensive) instruments and equipment that can measure dynamic acuity, peripheral awareness, and eye–hand and eye–foot coordination and collect other valuable data for the scientific tracking of sports vision training results. These data quantify vision training results in a way that cannot easily be done in the field and can prove the efficacy of *SportsVision* training. A well-equipped vision training clinic provides access to the lenses, prisms, and sophisticated electronic testing and training devices that cannot always be used outside of this environment.

Clinical training is not always feasible, however. In addition to the expense and time needed to attend clinical sessions, it is often impossible to get a player or an entire team to a laboratory to participate in a sports vision training program. Moreover, even the best lab setting cannot exactly replicate the playing field. Fortunately, though, you do not *need* a sophisticated clinical laboratory in order to practice *SportsVision* training.

While there are benefits to *SportsVision* training in a clinical setting, *SportsVision* training can also be done outside of the laboratory: at home, in the training area, or on the field or court. *SportsVision* training and evaluation can be done anywhere the athlete plays. However, this book is not intended to replace a complete vision laboratory and training program supervised by an experienced clinician. Ideally, for best results, an athlete should undertake a combination of specialized clinical testing and training as well as home- or field-based training.

Sports Vision Laboratory

A well-equipped sports vision clinical laboratory has myriad instruments to improve the athlete's visual skills. Much as a weight room offers equipment that is used to build the strength, muscular endurance, and power of an athlete, the sports vision laboratory offers equipment to train the athlete's visual system. In the laboratory, the principle of loading the visual system is frequently used. It is not uncommon

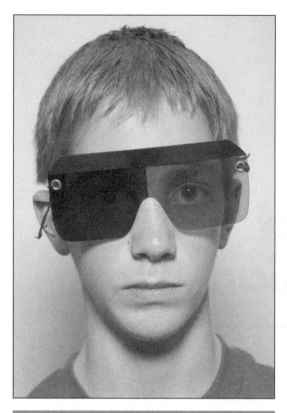

Figure 2.1 Red-green glasses used to enhance binocular vision performance.

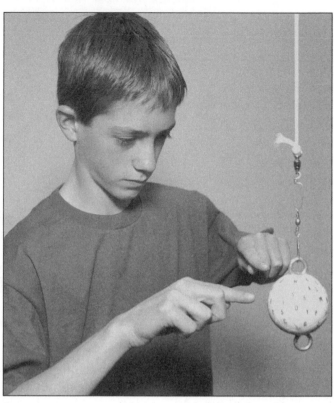

Figure 2.2 Athlete hitting a swinging VDP ball for eye–hand coordination.

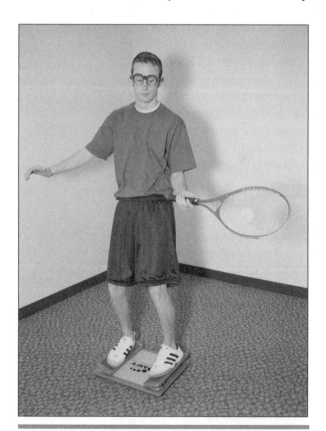

Figure 2.3 Loading the visual system with yoke prism glasses while balancing on an MFT device to enhance eye–foot coordination skills.

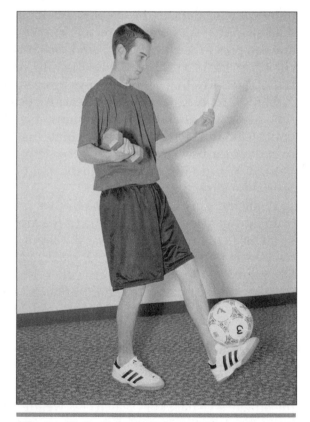

Figure 2.4 Enhancement of the vergence system through multiple loading exercises.

in a sports vision clinic to see an athlete wearing prism glasses and balancing on a balance beam while trying to catch a ball (figure 2.5). The idea is that by stressing or loading the visual system in a clinical *SportsVision* environment, athletes will be better able to perform under the actual stresses of their sport. In the sports vision laboratory, a training activity needs to simulate actual playing conditions as closely as possible. For example, rather than sitting down while performing a visual exercise, the athlete can dribble a soccer ball or move a hockey puck back and forth while performing the *SportsVision* exercise (figure 2.6). One of the advantages of *SportsVision* field training is that *SportsVision* sport conditions do not have to be simulated because *SportsVision* exercises can be done while performing actual sport skills. Chapter 5 provides sport-specific *SportsVision* training exercises and ways to modify them for field use.

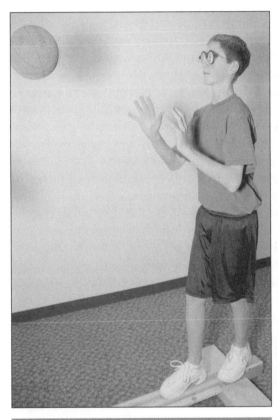

Figure 2.5   Athlete catching a ball while wearing prism glasses.

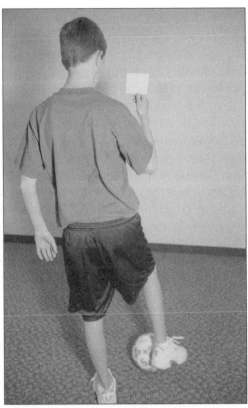

Figure 2.6   Making a vision therapy exercise a *SportsVision* exercise by using sport-specific equipment while performing the exercise.

In our *SportsVision* laboratory, we routinely provide seven weekly hour-long training sessions that include pre- and posttraining testing. This testing shows athletes how much they have improved over the course of the training sessions. During that seven-week training period, homework is always assigned. We ask the athlete to do at least 15 to 30 minutes of sport-specific *SportsVision* training on the field or in the training environment during each day of practice. We are often asked by coaches and athletes who routinely perform *SportsVision* training for additional work that they can do while not on the practice field. We provide home *SportsVision* activities for motivated athletes in chapter 5. However, we compared NCAA Division I athletes who did *SportsVision* training both at home and under a coach's supervision on the field and in practice with those who did similar exercises only at home with no supervision. We found that the athletes who were supervised on the field also did their home training exercises on a regular basis, whereas the athletes who had only a home program did not regularly complete these activities. This showed us that for best compliance with a home program, *SportsVision* training needs to be done both on the field or court and at home.

SportsVision Applications

For athletes and coaches who do not have access to a professional sports vision laboratory, many types of applied *SportsVision* training equipment are still available—some that is readily available in the coach's equipment bag. Creativity plays a large role in a successful *SportsVision* program, just as it does for successfully coaching *SportsVision*. Once you have completed reading this book, you will not be able to walk into a toy store or sporting goods store again without purchasing some new *SportsVision* training equipment! Chapter 3 discusses equipment in greater detail.

For a *SportsVision* training program to be most effective, it should incorporate the equipment that is customarily used in a particular sport. For example, youth soccer coaches can use cones and a soccer ball during sport-specific *SportsVision* activities. The coach can have athletes use peripheral awareness to detect objects that the coach holds up, such as different numbers of fingers or objects of different colors, while the athletes keep their heads up and dribble the ball during dribbling drills. A youth football coach can put numbers or letters on the football and have players look closely at the ball and call out as many numbers or letters as they can before making the catch in passing drills. The player who can identify the most characters while catching the ball wins the drill. This simple activity develops visual concentration, eye–hand coordination, and figure–ground responses. We provide numerous modifications of applied *SportsVision* exercises, but the variations of *SportsVision* training activities are limited only by the imagination of the coach, athlete, or parent.

High school, college, and professional athletes can also do *SportsVision* exercises while training in the weight room. Eye charts can be placed on the walls or ceiling around some of the benches, racks, or platforms to allow lifters to do eye tracking and eye movement skills while lifting. These activities can improve eye movement and accuracy while engaging in a stressful activity, but we do not recommend working on eye movement and accuracy skills while performing maximal lifts. It is more important to concentrate on the lift itself during 1RM to 3RM lifts. However, when the athlete lifts 6RM or lighter loads, working on eye movement and accuracy skills can improve the athlete's overall performance when faced with the extra load of the game. *SportsVision* exercises can be performed as part of a circuit weight-training program at supplemental stations. *SportsVision* exercises can also be performed by partners during rest intervals between sets or while waiting for access to a particular exercise station.

For offensive linemen in American football, mental, physical, and visual fatigue begin to set in toward the end of the third quarter as a result of the stress of blocking. It is not that the athlete cannot see, but as you learned in chapter 1, eye muscles can also fatigue under prolonged stress. By overloading both the visual system and the muscular system during resistance training, the athlete develops not only muscular strength and endurance but visual endurance as well. The lineman must also be able to focus on more than just the defender in front of him during each play. Working on eye movement and accuracy as well as peripheral awareness trains him to see more of the field and run or block passes more effectively. In a drill with NCAA Division I football linemen, we found that some of the linemen suppressed one eye while blocking. When the linemen hit a blocking sled, over 50 percent of them shut one eye because of the stress to the body. Suppressing one eye while blocking can result in not seeing a critical defender who is trying to sack the quarterback. During a six-week *SportsVision* training program, the linemen put on red-green glasses while viewing a red-green chart. One eye could see the green letters but not the red, and vice versa, much like reading a 3D comic book. After this training, none of the linemen suppressed either eye when hitting the blocking sled in the same drill.

Another weight room *SportsVision* activity is peripheral and central awareness training. When the body is placed under stress, sympathetic overload takes place. This tends to dilate the pupils as part of the fight or flight response of the sympathetic nervous system, resulting in more defocused and blurred vision. Training the system to be both peripherally and centrally aware under a sympathetic overload creates a much more efficient athlete. This training can be done in the weight room and on the field with a peripheral awareness chart (see appendix I.2). A peripheral awareness chart has a detailed central object on which the athlete focuses, and progressively larger numbers or shapes radiate out from the center. The athlete concentrates on the center object while trying to identify the peripheral objects. This can be done while undertaking a strenuous activity such as resistance training or a specific sport skill. Peripheral awareness can be trained through the exercises and modifications presented in chapters 4 and 5. To use the peripheral awareness chart in appendix I.2, place the chart approximately 12 inches from the athlete's face. Have the athlete concentrate on the central figure while identifying the peripheral letters

While on the field or court, athletes can easily engage in *SportsVision* training during warm-ups or during the rest interval between repetitions of a sport-specific skill drill. For example, when half the players on a soccer team are performing a drill, the players who are waiting can work on soccer-specific *SportsVision* training exercises rather than goof around. *SportsVision* exercises can provide effective training in a limited period of time. Creativity and variety in a training session yield the best results.

SportsVision exercises can be done while using any type of equipment for a given sport, including plyometric balls, large stabilization balls, blocking dummies, basketball backboards, volleyball or soccer nets, baseball gloves, and any type of goal used in a given sport. You can modify the sport-specific ball or equipment to enhance *SportsVision* training (see chapter 5). For example, you can use a marking pen to change the color of the seams of a tennis ball; this visual enhancement can help the player follow the ball to the racket.

Static Versus Dynamic *SportsVision* Training

Most sports vision clinics or labs use static vision enhancement training; vision training is done primarily in the clinic or lab. The athlete's responses to the training program and improvements in their static visual skills are closely monitored. These types of programs tend to be very clinical in nature and delivery. Visual improvements should translate to an improvement in athletic performance; the carryover to actual sport performance is better when the training more closely simulates actual sport situations. Dynamic *SportsVision* takes sports vision enhancement to the training environment, weight room, and field or court. This enables the coach and athlete to use practice and training time more efficiently. Doing *SportsVision* activities during practice time can more quickly reveal the areas in which the athlete has shortcomings in visual performance. Practicing *SportsVision* in a dynamic environment offers positive reinforcement for the coach and athlete as they see visual and sport skill improvement over time. In addition, due to the competitive nature of athletes, as one athlete's visual performance improves, her teammates will also strive to improve their visual performance. Dynamic *SportsVision* training is much more practical, stimulating, time efficient, and competitive than static sports vision training programs.

Dynamic *SportsVision* training exercises can be done while moving or simulating the movement patterns of a particular sport. There are very few instances in sport where the athlete is stationary, so why perform sports vision training while sitting still? When athletes move or work on balance while performing *SportsVision* training exercises, they enhance the sport specificity of their vision training (see figure 2.7).

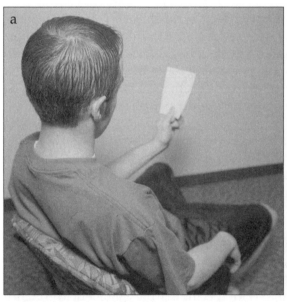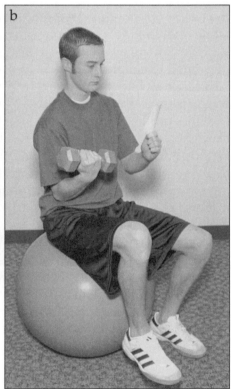

Figure 2.7 Training using a near–far chart while sitting *(a)* on a chair and *(b)* on a stabilization ball.

Relationship Between Balance and Vision

It has been estimated that over 20 percent of optic nerve fibers go to the balance centers of the cerebellum and cerebrum of the brain. To demonstrate the relationship between vision and balance, perform this simple exercise: Balance on one foot with your eyes open, and then close your eyes and try to continue balancing. Most people cannot maintain balance without falling to one side or touching the other foot to the ground. Balance is an integral part of every sport, and yet few coaches and athletes spend sufficient training time developing and improving dynamic balance for sport. *SportsVision* training can significantly enhance sport-specific dynamic balance. Almost every dynamic *SportsVision* training activity involves a balance component.

We classify balance activities in one of three categories: (1) generic balance, (2) sport-specific balance, and (3) *SportsVision* balance. A generic balance activity is a balance exercise in and of itself, whether it is done on a balance beam, with a tennis ball under each foot, sitting on a basketball with feet off the floor, in single-leg stance on the floor, on a mini trampoline, or using any other type of balance equipment. Sport-specific balance activities incorporate a sport-specific skill with the balance training, such as catching a ball while balancing on one foot on a balance beam, or volleying a soccer ball with one foot while the other foot is balancing on a mini trampoline. But to truly overload the balance systems, the athlete must do *SportsVision* balance training exercises. An example of a *SportsVision* balance exercise would be balancing on one foot on a balance beam and playing catch with a football; a wide receiver would also complete a visual tracing without dropping the ball or letting the nonsupporting foot touch the balance beam or the floor (see figure 2.8). This visual addition to the balance exercise heightens eye movement skills, peripheral awareness skills, eye–hand and eye–foot coordination, as well as balance skills. It is also a tremendous amount of fun and can be used to motivate players competitively.

SportsVision balance training can be accomplished on a variety of inexpensive balance devices. An athlete can simply use a two-inch-by-four-inch board that is two feet long. Performing *SportsVision* balance exercises on this board dramatically increases the challenge of the activity by placing a greater load on the athlete's visual system. Tennis balls, mini trampolines, balance beams, foam rolls, and large stabilization balls can all be used to train balance. Many other more expensive balance training

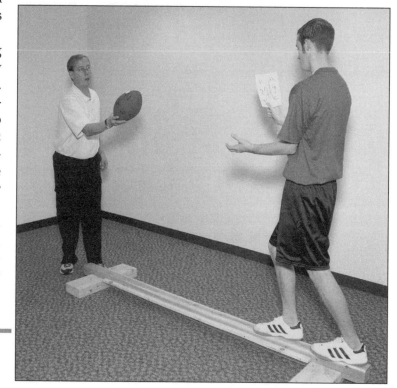

Figure 2.8 *SportsVision* balance exercise: doing visual tracings while playing catch.

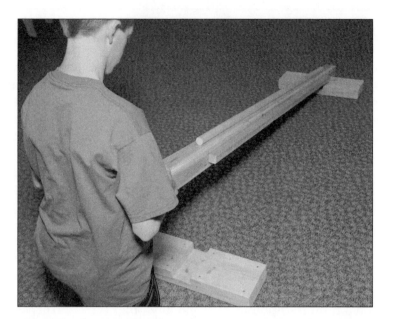

Figure 2.9   Four-in-one balance beam.

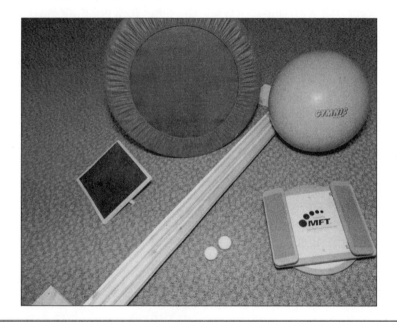

Figure 2.10   Balance apparatus.

devices are available, but their cost may be prohibitive. The four-in-one balance beam includes four different surfaces on which to perform dynamic balance (see figure 2.9; also see appendix A for information on constructing your own). A variety of sliding boards, used primarily by skiers, can be effectively used by almost any athlete. Figure 2.10 shows a variety of these balance devices.

When incorporating *SportsVision* into any athletic program, from youth leagues to professional sports, dynamic vision and balance should be addressed as part of every training session. Coaches frequently separate vision and balance training. However, the visual-vestibular system does not separate the two. Visual and vestibular interaction can be trained and enhanced game by game over the entire season. It does not take expensive equipment or additional training time; however, it does take creativity and an open mind to these new and exciting training procedures. Dynamic *SportsVision* training can be an enjoyable and fulfilling addition to the sometimes monotonous rigors of training. In the next few chapters, we discuss designing and executing a sport-specific *SportsVision* training program for athletes in a variety of sports.

Balance Training Equipment

Of all the loading activities we have described in *SportsVision*, balance is perhaps one of the most important, because of its direct correlation to sport performance. Of the 17 sports listed that have specific *SportsVision* training programs, every one requires tremendous balance to be successful. Therefore, a significant number of our training exercises use some aspect of balance as a method of loading.

One of our primary goals in presenting *SportsVision* is to provide a program that ANY athlete can use to improve his or her on-field abilities. To that end, we have tried to keep the cost of the loading equipments, as well as the testing and evaluation tools, to a minimum.

However, there are several pieces of equipment that are on the market today that provide excellent loading and balance demands or challenges to the *SportsVision* training exercises. This equipment can be purchased through one of several exercise and rehabilitative equipment vendors, such as Power Systems Sports, EFI, and Perform Better. We have included references for these companies in appendix F. Many athletic training rooms and weight rooms may already have some of these balance devices for use in the rehabilitation of athletic injuries, or as part of a sport-specific resistance training program. The MFT (My Function Trainer), the BAPS (Biomechanical Ankle Platform System) board, the Fitter, the Body Blade, and a host of other balance devices can easily be incorporated into any *SportsVision* exercise modification during the 30-day training period. For the most part, these types of balance devices are more sport specific, and consequently, tend to be more advanced than the simple two-by-four, teeter board, or balance beam. If the athlete has easy access to one or more of these excellent pieces of equipment, we encourage them to utilize those devices during their *SportsVision* training.

Chapter ③

Designing a *SportsVision* Program

A major league baseball first baseman came to us several years ago to have a sport-specific *SportsVision* program designed for him. This athlete wanted to improve his eye–hand coordination, peripheral awareness, and balance to increase his batting average and fielding percentage over the previous season. His goal was to hit over .300 and reduce his fielding errors. He worked diligently over the off-season on his *SportsVision* training exercises with the same intensity he had in the weight room. In fact, our staff could always tell when he was in the clinic because they could smell the sweat he produced because of how hard he was training while doing his vision exercises. The year after starting his vision training, he achieved his own personal-best batting average, .327. Unfortunately, that was the last year of his professional career due to an accident that forced him to retire from baseball. However, he still thanks us for that great season and all that *SportsVision* did to improve his game.

This chapter discusses the basics of designing a *SportsVision* training program. As for any sport-specific training program, several factors need to be considered in order to make the program most effective. To evaluate the efficacy of *SportsVision* training, it is necessary to evaluate the athlete's visual skills before and after training. This can be accomplished two ways. First, if the coach or athlete has access to a sports vision facility, a professional can do the evaluation. However, if the coach or athlete does not have access to this type of facility, with minimal equipment and the evaluation form provided in appendix B, a very effective *SportsVision* evaluation can be done.

Athletes frequently request normative data after testing to see how they compare with other athletes. An average score is provided for each evaluation for such comparisons. It should be noted that visual performance varies greatly from athlete to athlete and sport to sport. Coaches may find that a particular athlete scores very high on certain tests while other athletes struggle with the same evaluation. The most important comparison is the pre- to posttraining changes for each athlete.

It is not uncommon for athletes to gravitate to a particular sport or position based on their physical and visual capabilities. By improving visual skills, athletes can also expand their possibilities in their sport. For example, one of our youth soccer players was traditionally a forward and played at the highest level in this position. Despite her success, she missed many scoring opportunities. When an outside midfield player was needed for the remainder of the season due to an injury, this athlete volunteered to play outside and had the best season of her career to date. She scored the most goals and became one of the best midfield players in the state. During our *SportsVision* evaluation of this player, we found she had poor directionality and decreased peripheral awareness, which decreased her effectiveness in the forward position, for which directionality and peripheral awareness are critical to success. As a midfield player, her directionality limitations were counteracted by playing primarily on the right side of the field. During the off-season, we gave her a *SportsVision* training program for soccer, as outlined in chapter 5, along with special exercises to address her weaknesses. She was able to return to the forward position in the next season and had much greater success than in previous seasons.

Pre- and Posttraining *SportsVision* Evaluation

It is our philosophy that athletes should be tested as they are trained and trained as they are tested. Thus, all the *SportsVision* evaluation tests are also found as training exercises in chapter 4. During evaluation, none of the suggestions for loading should be used. The *SportsVision* evaluation is the same for all sports and positions. Just as a 40-yard dash can be used to test any athlete's sprint speed, the same tests are used for all athletes in the basic *SportsVision* evaluation. Six tests of basic visual skills make up the *SportsVision* evaluation. The same form is used for both pretraining and posttraining evaluations. The following sections give an explanation of each *SportsVision* test procedure.

Focusing

The near–far chart, exercise 3 in chapter 4 (page 40), tests focusing abilities (see figure 3.1). This test assesses flexibility and speed of the focusing system. The materials needed are a stopwatch, a small letter chart, and a large letter chart (these charts appear in appendixes I.3 and I.4). Place the large letter chart on a wall at the farthest point where the athlete can still clearly read the letters. Hold the small letter chart approximately four inches from the athlete's face at nose level. Have the athlete read the letters from left to right, alternating from the near chart to the far chart. Count the number of letters that the athlete reads in one minute, and record that number. Perform the test three times, and average the scores. A typical score is between 60 and 70 letters read per minute.

Tracking

The two-strip saccades, exercise 6 in chapter 4 (page 42), test tracking ability (see figure 3.2). Saccadic tracking is the ability of the eyes to quickly and accurately jump from point to point in space. You need two letter strips (which appear in appendixes I.6, I.7, and I.8) and a stopwatch. Attach the two strips to a wall three feet apart, and have the athlete stand at arm's length from the wall. Instruct the athlete to keep her head still while performing the test. Have the athlete start at the upper left-hand column of the charts and then alternate reading letters from column to column. Upon reaching the bottom of the first columns, the athlete should alternate from chart to chart down the second columns. Continue this procedure for one minute. The score is the number of letters read in this time. Repeat three times, and average the three scores. A typical score is between 60 and 70 letters per minute.

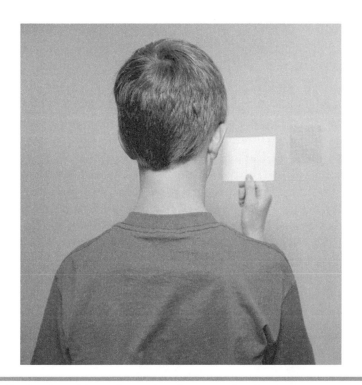

Figure 3.1 Evaluation of focusing using the near–far chart test.

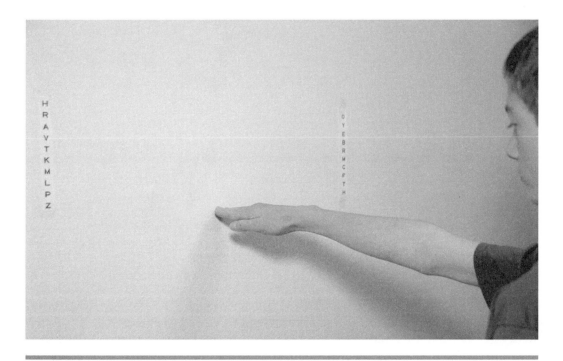

Figure 3.2 Evaluation of tracking using the two-strip saccades test.

Vergence

Pencil push-ups, exercise 20 in chapter 4 (page 54), test vergence skills (see figure 3.3). Vergence is the ability to accurately cross and uncross the eyes, which allows the athlete to maintain single (binocular) vision from near to far and from far to near. The materials needed are a pencil or pen and a tape measure. The coach or assistant tells the athlete to keep his head still. The coach or assistant holds the pencil, with the tip pointing up, approximately two feet in front of the athlete's nose. The coach or assistant slowly moves the pencil toward the athlete's nose, asking him to call out when he sees two pencil tips. At that point, measure and record the distance from the tip of the pencil to the athlete's nose. Repeat three times, and average the three scores. A typical score is zero to two inches; most athletes should be able to avoid double vision until the pencil tip reaches their nose.

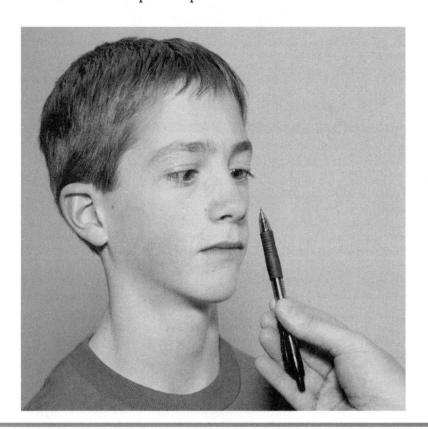

Figure 3.3 Evaluation of vergence using pencil push-ups.

Sequencing

Hand sequencing, exercise 22 in chapter 4 (page 56), tests sequencing, the ability to organize visual information in a given order. Sequencing helps the athlete organize instructions, plays, and events during the game. The only material needed is a sequencing form for the coach (given in appendix C). The sequencing form lists the letters P, S, and F in random order. The letters indicate a hand position: P means palm down on the table, S means the side of the hand down on the table, and F means fist on the table. The coach or assistant sits at a table, directly across from the athlete, and performs a series of hand movements. The coach starts with a sequence of 3 movements and adds one movement each time, up to 10 movements. The athlete repeats the same sequence of hand movements (see figure 3.4). The score is the largest sequence completed correctly. Repeat the test three times. The coach can change of the order of the sequence in subsequent trials. Average the three scores. A typical score is approximately 6 to 8.

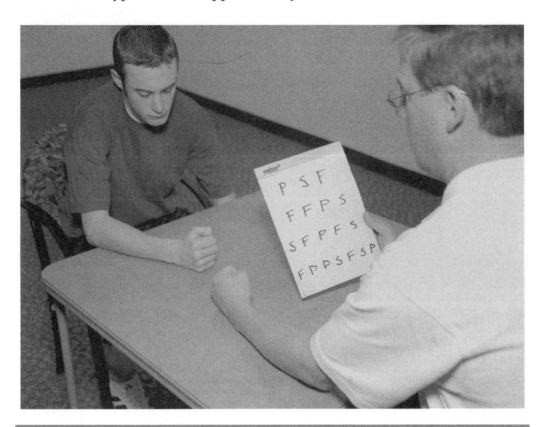

Figure 3.4   Evaluation of sequencing using the hand sequencing test.

Eye-Hand Coordination

Use the egg carton catch, exercise 38 in chapter 4 (page 68), to test eye–hand coordination (figure 3.5). Materials needed for this test are an empty 12-egg carton or container, a quarter, a marking pen, and a stopwatch. Write the number 1 in the upper left egg holder of the egg carton, the number 2 in the egg holder below that (the lower left corner), and follow that sequence until the number 12 is in the lower right corner of the egg container. Place the quarter in the number 1 holder. The athlete stands holding the egg carton at a comfortable level. The athlete holds the lid open and flips the quarter sequentially from compartment number 1 to 2 and so on up to number 12. If the quarter falls out of the egg carton or lands in the wrong number, the athlete must replace the quarter in the last compartment correctly completed and continue from there. Time how long it takes the athlete to get the quarter to the number 12 compartment. Repeat three times, and average the three scores (in seconds). A typical score is 15 to 20 seconds to complete 12 sequential flips.

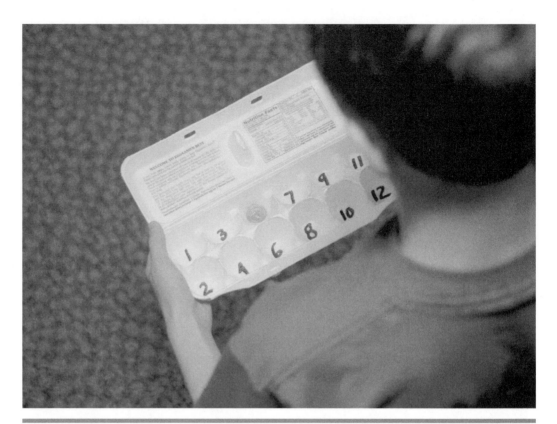

Figure 3.5 Evaluation of eye–hand coordination using the egg carton catch.

Visualization

The last test in the *SportsVision* evaluation is Ace to Seven, adapted from exercise 45 in chapter 4 (page 76). Visualization is the ability to "see" an image or scene in the mind's eye. The materials needed are a deck of cards and a stopwatch. The coach puts the seven cards from ace to seven of the same suit in random order on a table. The coach starts the watch as soon as all the cards are presented face up to the athlete. The athlete studies the cards for as long as needed to memorize the order of the cards. The timer is running while the athlete is memorizing the order. Once the athlete feels ready, the athlete turns the cards face down, from left to right (see figure 3.6). The athlete turns the cards up in order from ace to seven; stop the timer when all cards are turned over in the correct sequence. If a card is turned out of sequence, the athlete must turn all cards face down and start again. Repeat three times, and average the three scores. A typical score is approximately 60 seconds.

The final section of chapter 4 gives exercises to improve directionality. This visual motor skill is not included in the evaluation process because it is too difficult to quantify accurately. However, all athletes should review this section to train and have fun with those *SportsVision* exercises as well.

Setting Up the Program

After completing the pretraining evaluation, you can design an appropriate *SportsVision* training program. A *SportsVision* training program should include two components: exercises to address any visual deficits as determined by the evaluation and the specific *SportsVision* exercises for your sport, given in chapter 5. If a deficit has been identified, numerous exercises to improve specific visual skills are given in chapter 4. Athletes should try all the exercises in chapter 4 that address their particular deficits to find the exercises that challenge them and offer them the most benefit. After mastering a basic exercise, athletes can try the suggestions for loading for that exercise to further improve their visual and motor skills. After a six-week training period, a post-training evaluation can assess the efficacy of the *SportsVision* training. Coaches and athletes will be amazed at the improvement in performance if they are as dedicated to their *SportsVision* training as they are to the other aspects of their training.

To conduct a *SportsVision* training program, the necessary equipment for conducting *SportsVision* exercises needs to be considered. While some professional facilities have sophisticated computers, lenses, prisms, and other expensive equipment, it is our intention to bring *SportsVision* to every coach and athlete. Therefore, all the equipment needed for the exercises in this book either can be purchased at local toy stores or sporting goods stores or on the Internet or can be made with our instructions by the coach or athlete. *SportsVision* equipment is discussed later in this chapter.

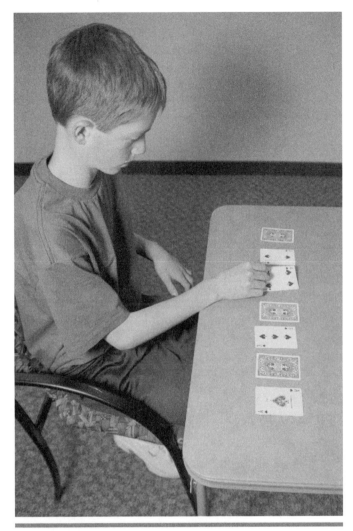

Figure 3.6 Evaluation of visualization using the Ace to Seven test.

An important variable in the design of the *SportsVision* training program is loading. In *SportsVision* training, loading is the process of making a particular task or exercise more difficult by adding motor skills or visual activities. For example, riding a bicycle is initially a very difficult motor task. Many learners practice with training wheels to assist with balance, and then one training wheel and then the other is removed. After more practice, elaborate and complex tricks can be added, as seen in competitive BMX and trick riding. When these riders simply ride their bicycles to the track, that once difficult task is now completely effortless. Similarly, many athletes initially struggle with the *SportsVision* exercises in chapter 4. With time, practice, and loading, athletes can become extremely proficient at specific visual skills.

Loading activities in *SportsVision* training follow the same principle that applies to all sports conditioning and training: the principle of specific adaptations to imposed demands (SAID; i.e., the body will adapt to the specific demands of training). Loading is the single factor that separates a basic visual exercise program from a *SportsVision* program. Additionally loaded activities should be considered only after a basic exercise has been mastered.

In an interview during Monday Night Football in the fall 2002 season, Donovan McNabb, the quarterback for the Philadelphia Eagles, talked about using strobe glasses while he was practicing. These loading devices decrease the amount of time that the athlete sees the target or opponents. McNabb was practicing his job in darkness approximately 50 percent of the time. This requires a heightened visual awareness that carries over to normal playing conditions. McNabb commented that after he removed the strobe glasses, everyone seemed to be running in slow motion, and he felt he had much more time to find the receiver and avoid the defenders. This is the essence of loading the visual system. The strobe glasses Donovan McNabb uses are fairly expensive. This book can give any athlete the same experience that McNabb feels after wearing the strobe glasses, but at a fraction of the cost.

SportsVision Equipment

To make *SportsVision* training available to every athlete, we include tests and exercises that require minimal equipment or equipment that is readily available to most athletes. In many cases, we present instructions in the appendixes for making the *SportsVision* training equipment used in this book. For example, the suggestions for loading the exercises in chapter 4 include numerous common types of balance apparatus. The mini trampoline and the large exercise or balance ball are the only pieces of equipment that cost a significant amount. However, foam rolls, a balance board, or other types of balance device can easily be substituted for the listed apparatus.

Sport-specific equipment can be modified for *SportsVision* training with some form of marking (figure 3.7). For example, the seams of a tennis ball can be marked

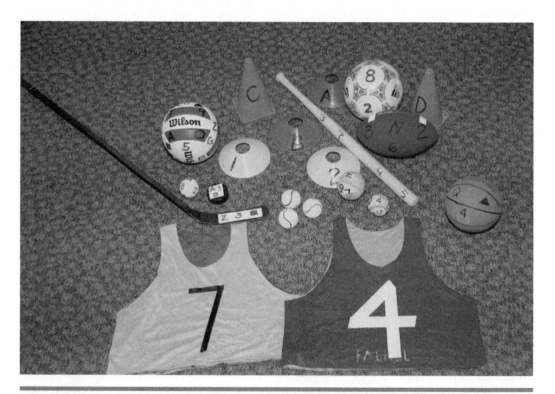

Figure 3.7 Sport-specific equipment modified for *SportsVision* training exercises. By simply placing numbers, letters, or shapes on any sport equipment, the coach can make any fundamental skill or game more challenging.

a color that contrasts with the ball to assist the tennis player in visually tracking and following the ball to the racket face. The same can be done with a softball or baseball for hitters, a football for wide receivers, and so on. A soccer ball can be marked with several different numbers and letters to help players watch the ball as they learn to head it or to kick it with spin. A volleyball can also be marked with numbers, letters, or shapes that players must call out before setting or spiking the ball. Number or letter charts can be placed on the backboard for basketball players to use in some *SportsVision* activities while shooting the basketball. The coach can place numbers on cones that are used to mark the field and have athletes find a particular numbered cone on the field. None of these sport-specific *SportsVision* techniques has any additional cost but enhances athletes' sports vision skills and abilities.

There is no limit to the types of equipment that can be used for *SportsVision* training. One of the best places to get *SportsVision* training equipment is a local toy store. A Frisbee® marked with numbers or letters can enhance dynamic acuity when athletes call out the characters before catching it. Nerf® paddle sets can be used with multiple balls while athletes balance on a balancing device or use a strobe light. In addition, many games in most toy stores promote visual perceptual awareness. For example, the coach can hold an I SPY® book in front of two athletes and have them spy the different objects requested at the bottom of the page or rotate the book to enhance their figure–ground perception and dynamic acuity in a fun and interactive way. The old classic Operation® game can be used to improve eye–hand coordination by having athletes play with their nondominant hand, while balancing, while moving their head, or a variety of other loading techniques. We enjoy seeing how many different modifications of our *SportsVision* exercises athletes and coaches can come up with. We are always fascinated with the endless possibilities for *SportsVision* training exercises.

Tach Targets

One of the most important aspects of sport but one that is rarely trained is field or court awareness. How many times do coaches wish that their athletes would look up and see their surroundings during the game? How many times has an athlete been frustrated by not getting the ball when she was wide open? The best athletes are able to perform multiple tasks simultaneously during the game. Most coaches assume that this valuable skill is an innate gift that an athlete either possesses or doesn't, but it is easy to train this skill. Training devices called tach targets help develop field or court awareness. Appendix H has a number of tach targets, which are different colors, shapes, arrows, letters, and so on that can be held up by the coach or assistant while the athletes are involved in skill development or practices on the field or court. An athlete can look for a tach target or find an unmarked player while trying to retain control of the ball or pass the ball to a teammate in a practice. These drills teach them better field or court awareness in actual competition. Using tach targets in practice leads to more attentive and coachable players in games. Players who can readily find tach targets during practice can hear the coach's comments or see the coach's signals without interrupting their play or their focus on the game.

Vision → Decision → Precision

When athletes have better visual skills, they can make faster and better decisions. If they have the time to make multiple decisions, they can more precisely implement those decisions and thus be more successful. We call this chain of events vision → decision → precision (VDP). It is this fundamental principle that underlies *SportsVision* training.

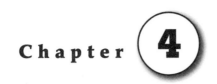

Chapter **4**

SportsVision Training Exercises

Now, let the fun begin! In this chapter, we present 50 *SportsVision* training exercises. These exercises are grouped by the visual motor or visual perceptual skill that they primarily develop. In addition, for most of the exercises, we give suggestions for loading to make them more difficult and challenging. Note that these loading exercises carefully take into account the specific skill being trained. Loading activities should be added only after the specific basic exercise has been mastered. However, these loading suggestions can be creatively augmented by the coach or athlete. Loading is an important factor that separates a basic visual training program from a *SportsVision* program.

Loading

The following loading techniques can be used to enhance the *SportsVision* exercises described in this chapter.

Balance

Figure 4.1, *a* through *g*, shows seven different balance adaptations:

a. Single-foot balance
b. Teeter board
c. Four-in-one balance beam
d. Tennis balls
e. Mini trampoline
f. Balance ball
g. 2" × 4" balance board

Because balance is such an integral component of all sport skills and of sports vision enhancement, balance activities constitute most loading exercises. The goal of all balance activities is to perfect the vision exercise while maintaining balance and body control. Athletes should strive to simulate the type of balance required for their sport whenever possible. Balance activities on the teeter board, four-in-one balance beam, tennis balls, and mini trampoline can be accomplished first with two feet on the apparatus (one foot on each tennis ball) and can progress to single-foot

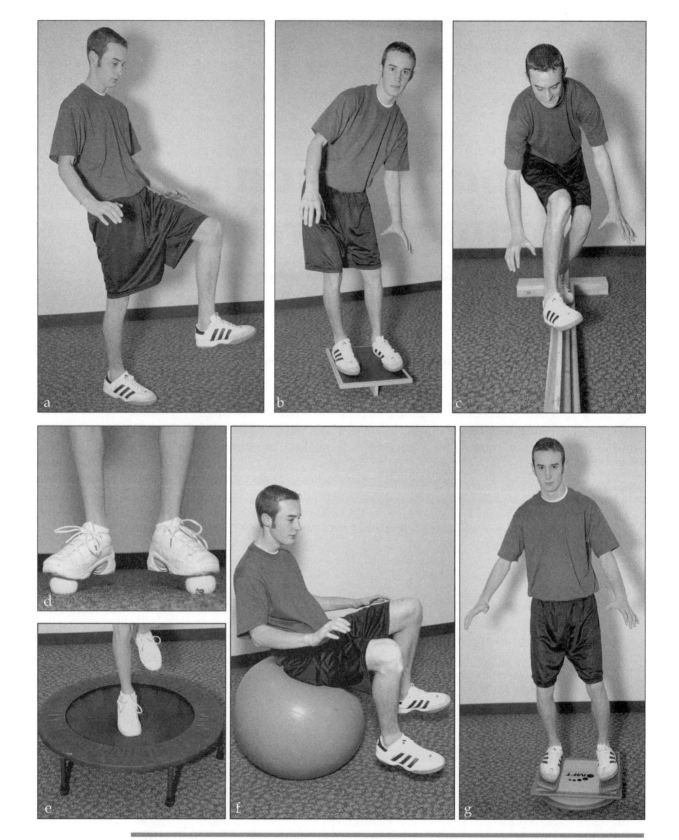

Figure 4.1 *(a)* Single-foot balance. *(b)* Teeter board. *(c)* Four-in-one balance beam. *(d)* Balancing on tennis balls. *(e)* Mini trampoline. *(f)* Balance ball. *(g)* MFT balance board.

balance on each piece of balance equipment as skill improves. The balance ball is used primarily during sitting exercises, progressing from two-foot to one-foot to no-foot support as balance improves. The athlete should always use two-foot support on the balance board.

Appendix A describes how to construct the four-in-one balance beam. Appendix D describes how to construct a teeter board. A 2" × 4" balance board can be purchased from EFI (see appendix F).

Juggling

For juggling as a loading activity, use three beanbags of equal weight. Depending on the skill and motivation of the athletes, various other items can be juggled for different degrees of difficulty, such as tennis balls, sport-specific balls (e.g., baseballs, softballs, footballs, basketballs, volleyballs), or three different types of balls.

One Eye Open (Monocular Vision)

To keep only one eye open as a way to load an exercise, the athlete cannot cover the other eye with the hand because most exercises require both hands. Therefore, have the athlete simply close one eye voluntarily.

Resistance Exercises

For many of the exercises, loading can be achieved by using dumbbells, medicine balls, or elastic tubing for simultaneous resistance work. The coach should use discretion when using resistance activities for loading, and maximal resistance should not be used when performing *SportsVision* exercises. Spotting may be appropriate during resistance-loaded activities.

Gaze Work

There are very few times in sport when an athlete looks directly straight ahead. Therefore, many *SportsVision* exercises should be performed in various positions of gaze, as discussed in chapter 1 and illustrated in figure 1.3. For the greatest sport specificity, a basketball player should perform many of the *SportsVision* exercises in superior gaze, for instance, whereas the hockey player should perform many of the *SportsVision* exercises in inferior gaze.

Head Movements

Many exercises are more difficult when a slow clockwise or counterclockwise movement of the head is performed. This is very similar to gaze work, because the gaze of the athlete is continually changed by the rotation of the head. Such head movement is very common in most sports, and adding head movements to the exercises dramatically assists the athlete with field awareness.

Motor Skills

Motor skills are the main activity of sports in general; therefore, adding these skills to *SportsVision* training simulates a realistic sport situation environment. The more athletes practice motor skills while simultaneously developing visual skills, the better prepared they will be for the stress of actual competition. The following five motor activities are used most often because they represent skills used in most sports. Coaches and athletes are encouraged to try other more sport-specific motor skills as athletes improve their sports vision skills.

a. Jumping jacks
b. Squats (without resistance)
c. Lunges
d. Abdominal exercises
e. Jogging in place

Metronome

Many of the exercises are greatly enhanced by adding the auditory stimulus of a metronome. This auditory stimulus is very beneficial in visual-sensory integration. The metronome sets the pace of a given exercise, from a very slow rhythm to a very fast, almost impossible, pace. A metronome can be purchased from any musical instrument dealer.

Strobe Light

Strobe work presents the athlete with a lighted stimulus for a very short period of time. Varying the frequency and duration of the light makes the visual exercises more difficult, as the object of concern is exposed to the retina for less time. This form of loading requires significantly heightened visual awareness, which can be extremely beneficial to an athlete's ability to concentrate under duress. Strobe activities should not be used until the athlete has mastered a particular exercise. Some activities, for example, playing catch with a strobe light in a dark room, can cause serious injury if the athlete is not extremely proficient. When using a strobe light for loading during catching exercises, athletes should generally start out using a beanbag and progress to their sport-specific implements only after becoming proficient under the strobe condition.

Plyometrics

Plyometric activities can be incorporated into *SportsVision* training. However, we do not recommend using box jumps, depth jumps, or other more advanced plyometric training stimuli while performing *SportsVision* exercises. Simple activities such as jumps in place, standing jumps, multiple jumps, and bounding can safely be performed while doing *SportsVision* training.

Many of the following exercises use special letter or number charts. These are included in the appendixes. Feel free to modify these charts to meet your needs.

In the next chapter, we modify these exercises for specific sports.

Focusing Exercises

Focusing is the ability to quickly, easily, and accurately perform near–far activities where the eyes are looking from a near point to a far point. This skill is necessary for a player to pay attention to a specific object or area in space. Training the focusing system can help the athlete perform difficult visual tasks with less visual fatigue.

1. Focusing Pursuits

Purpose   To improve eye movement and focusing skills

Materials   Three-by-five-inch card with 25 random letters and numbers on it in five rows by five columns

Procedure

1. The coach or athlete holds the card approximately 14 inches in front of the athlete's eyes, with the letters facing the athlete.

2. Slowly move the letter card in a circle in a plane parallel to the athlete's face, first closer and then farther away. The athlete tries to maintain the clarity of the letters while the card is moving. If the letters become blurry, slow down the movement until the athlete can keep them in focus.

3. Move the card in a horizontal or vertical oval. Also move the card above and below eye level.

4. The athlete's head should not move during the exercise.

Questions for the Athlete

• Is it more difficult as the card moves faster?

• Did you improve so that you could keep the letters clear even as the card moved faster?

• Was it easier to move your eyes in any particular pattern?

• Was it harder when the letters were closer or farther away?

• Did you feel your eyes moving?

• Did you feel your eyes focusing?

Signs of Improvement   Ability to increase rotational speed while keeping letters in focus

Suggestions for Loading

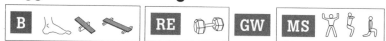

2. Near–Far Eye Jumps

Purpose   To change focus quickly and accurately from a near point to a far point

Materials   Two targets (use sport-specific targets, e.g., two baseballs, two tennis balls)

Procedure

1. Place one target four inches or less away.

2. Place the second target 2 to 10 feet away.

3. The athlete looks at the near target, then the far target, and back to the near target. Be sure both eyes come into focus on the near target and diverge when looking at the far target.

4. Do 30 to 40 near–far eye jumps each day, or repeat for three to five minutes each day.

Signs of Improvement

- Ability to change from near to far target quickly and accurately
- Smooth eye movements

Suggestions for Loading

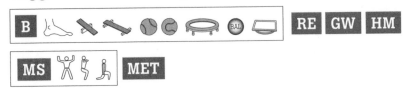

3. Near-Far Chart

Purpose

1. To improve the flexibility of the focusing system
2. To improve the ability to maintain clear vision at near and far distances

Materials

1. Small letter chart (appendix I.3)
2. Large letter chart (appendix I.4)

Procedure

1. Place the large letter chart on the wall at the farthest point where the athlete can still clearly read the letters.
2. Hold the small letter chart four inches from athlete's face at nose level.
3. The athlete reads letters from left to right, alternating between the near chart and the far chart.

Signs of Improvement

- Ability to see letters clearly on both near and far charts
- Ability to call letters in a steady rhythm without losing place
- Increased speed and accuracy over time

Suggestions for Loading

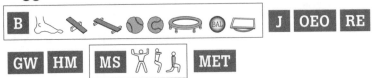

Tracking Exercises

Visual motor control requires the coordination of the 12 eye muscles (6 in each eye). This control lays the foundation for concentration, endurance, and visual efficiency. Tracking improves the eye's ability to stay on a target. Efficient tracking is the skill of smoothly, accurately, and attentively following a moving object. The bead string, exercise 9, is classically considered a vergence exercise, but because its fundamental basis is tracking, we have put it in this section. It can be used as either a tracking or vergence exercise.

4. Dice Pursuits

Purpose   To increase the ability to move the eyes accurately while performing a thinking task

Materials   One die

Procedure

1. The coach or a partner holds the die in front of the athlete's face and moves it slowly and smoothly in a random, unpredictable motion.
2. The athlete calls out the number showing.
3. While the die is still moving, the coach calls out an arithmetic problem (addition, subtraction, multiplication, or division) and rotates the die to a new number.
4. The athlete calls out the number showing on the die, solves the arithmetic problem, and then gives the answer while keeping his eyes on the moving die.
5. The answer to the arithmetic problem becomes the first number of the next problem.

Variation

• Start the exercise with relatively slow movement and easy arithmetic problems, and increase the speed and complexity as you go.

Signs of Improvement

• Ability to follow the die smoothly and accurately for longer periods of time
• Ability to perform mental arithmetic problems of increasing difficulty and increasing length without error

Suggestions for Loading

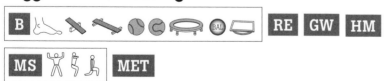

5. Find the Number

Purpose   To improve accuracy of eye movements and visual organization

Materials   Random number chart (appendix I.5) and a stopwatch

Procedure

1. The coach or a partner writes the numbers 1 through 20 on a piece of paper (see appendix I.5). The numbers should be written as large as possible.

2. The coach or a partner stands three to four feet away from the athlete, holding the numbered paper at chest level. The athlete stands with good posture where he can see the paper.

3. The coach or a partner tells the athlete to focus on one of the numbers on the paper. Then the coach asks the athlete to find another number on the paper, while the coach or partner monitors the athlete's eye movement as he scans the paper to find the next number requested.

4. Continue through all the numbers in either random order, or sequentially from one to twenty or twenty to one. Assess how long it takes for the athlete to complete the activity. The coach can also ask the athlete to perform simple mental arithmetic problems (e.g., 5 + 11 = 16), and scan for the correct answer (e.g., 16, in the example).

5. The coach constantly evaluates the athlete's ability and sets the tempo accordingly. It should be fast enough to be a challenge but slow enough to allow success. Tapping often helps establish the rhythm for the athlete.

6. Once the athlete becomes proficient at finding the requested number, the coach can further challenge the athlete by moving the paper in circular, "figure 8," or back and forth motions.

Signs of Improvement

1. Completion of the activity in less time

2. Improved performance while the coach or partner increases the activity's challenge by moving the paper faster

Suggestions for Loading

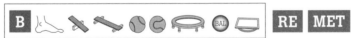

6. Two-Strip Saccades

Purpose   To increase speed and accuracy of saccades, or point-to-point eye movements

Materials

1. Three two-strip letter charts (appendixes I.6, I.7, and I.8)

2. Stopwatch

Procedure

1. Cut the two-strip letter chart down the middle. The fewer letters on a chart, the easier it is to complete this exercise. Start with the easiest chart and progress to the more difficult ones as tolerated.
2. Attach the two strips to the wall three feet apart.
3. The athlete stands at arm's length from the strips.
4. While holding his head still, the athlete reads the letters from left to right, alternating from chart to chart, down the columns.
5. As the athlete becomes proficient, vary the distance between the letter strips. The farther apart the letter strips are, the more difficult the activity.

Signs of Improvement

- Ability to read down the columns without losing one's place
- Ability to read down the columns with increasing speed
- Ability to progress to appendix I.7 and then appendix I.8

Suggestions for Loading

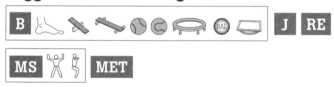

7. Ball Batting

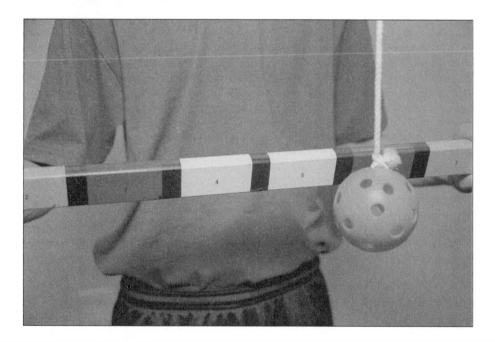

Figure 4.2   Ball batting.

Purpose   To coordinate eye movements and motor responses while attending to directions

Materials

1. Sport-appropriate bat, stick, or racket with number markings. Be creative in placing the numbers. They can be put on the handle, the webbing of the racket, the "sweet spot" of the bat, and so on. The numbers can be of various sizes and colors but should not be too small.

2. Ball suspended from a string

Procedure

1. The athlete holds the implement horizontally with one hand on each end so that numbers are facing her.

2. The coach or partner holds the string with the ball attached approximately three feet away from the athlete so it is at her chest level. As the coach or a partner calls out a number, the athlete hits the ball with the appropriate part of the implement.

3. The athlete continues hitting the ball, maintaining a steady rhythm, until a new number is called. The athlete then begins to hit the ball with the newly named part of the implement.

4. The athlete should hold her head still and locate proper point on the implement by moving the eyes only.

Signs of Improvement

- Smooth, accurate transitions to appropriate points on the implement
- Ability to locate proper points on the implement and to follow the path of the ball without head movement

Suggestions for Loading

B 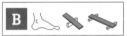   MET SL

8. Ball Tap

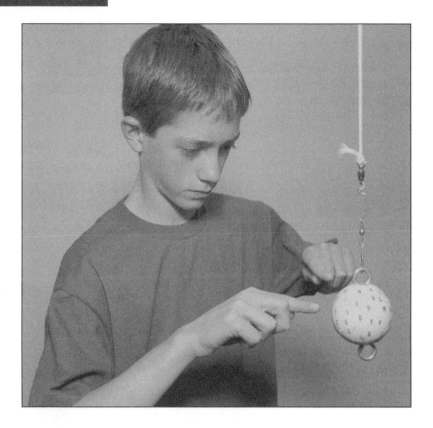

Figure 4.3 Ball tap.

Purpose To improve tracking abilities in association with motor responses

Materials Ball on an adjustable string approximately five feet long

Procedure

1. The coach or a partner holds the string so that the ball is located one to two feet away from the athlete at eye level. The athlete begins by tapping the ball lightly in a regular rhythm with his dominant hand.

2. Then the athlete taps ball with alternate hands, maintaining a steady rhythm (see figure 4.3).

3. Next, the athlete taps ball with just one finger, again beginning with the dominant hand and then alternating left and right.

4. If the activity is too difficult, start with larger ball and then progress to a smaller one.

5. Vary the height of the ball, and repeat steps 1 through 3.

Signs of Improvement

- Ability to follow the path of the ball with the eyes only, keeping the head still
- Ability to keep the ball going at a steady pace
- Ability to aim the ball at a specific target in space

Suggestions for Loading

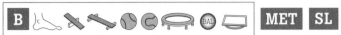

9. Bead String

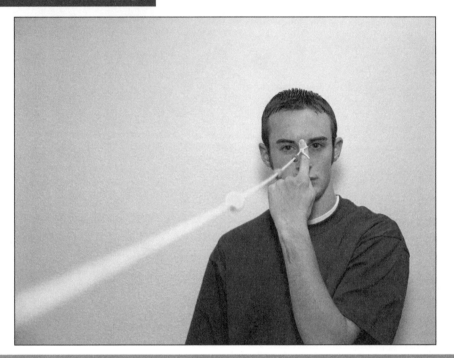

Figure 4.4   Bead string exercise.

Purpose

1. To develop the ability to perceive images from both eyes at the same time
2. To develop the ability to shift fixation quickly and accurately from one point to another

Materials   A 10-foot-long string with three wooden beads of different colors along it. The length of string can vary, based on the sport-specific training application (e.g., 60 feet, 6 inches for baseball players, the distance from foul line to backboard for basketball players). The beads should be approximately one-half inch in diameter. The beads should fit snuggly on the string so that they stay in place during this exercise. One end of the string is attached to an object, and the athlete holds the other end so that the string is taut.

Procedure

1. Position the beads along the string.
2. The athlete holds one end of the string taut with one finger between her eyes.
3. The athlete picks one bead to focus on and tries to see two strings going to the bead and crossing at the bead to make an X (see figure 4.4). Focusing at the last bead should form a V.
4. The athlete's eyes jump from bead to bead, maintaining awareness of two strings crossing at whichever bead is in view.

Signs of Improvement

- Ability to see two strings appearing to cross at the bead in focus
- Ability to maintain the center of the X on each bead while shifting from one bead to another

Suggestions for Loading

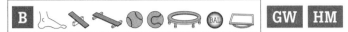

10. Double Bead String Fixations

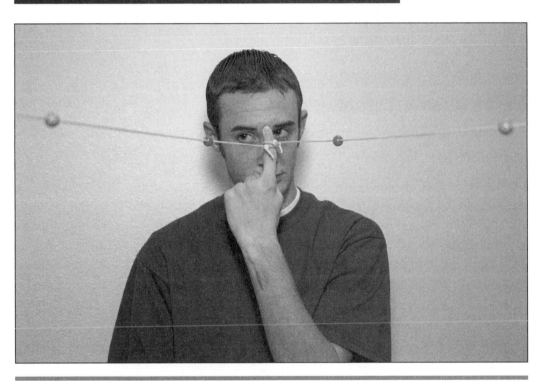

Figure 4.5 Double bead string fixation exercise. Note the athlete's extreme gaze position in this exercise.

Purpose   To improve accuracy and coordination of eye movement

Materials   Two 3- to 60-foot-long bead strings with two beads on each string, with one end attached to a wall or locker. The strings are attached to the wall or locker about one foot apart and about six inches below eye level.

Procedure

1. The athlete stands holding the ends of both strings taut on the tip of his nose.
2. The coach or a partner instructs the athlete as follows: 'Look at the left bead. Be aware of the rest of the room. Hold the X for a count of 4. Then look at the end of the string, be aware of the V, and hold the V for a count of 4.' The athlete should be familiar with exercise 9 so as to understand the X and V appearance of the string.
3. Repeat step 2 with the right bead and the right end of the string.

Variations

- Have the athlete change fixation on command.
- Vary the position of the beads.

Signs of Improvement   Increased speed and accuracy of eye movement over time

Suggestions for Loading

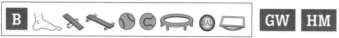

Comments   This is a great warm-up activity before going out onto the field for an athletic event because it works on speed and accuracy of eye movements with minimal equipment and in minimal space. The two bead strings can be attached to the athlete's locker.

11. Flashlight Chase

Purpose   To integrate eye movement and motor response in all regions of gaze

Materials   Two flashlights

Procedure

1. Work in a darkened room on a large, blank wall if possible.
2. The coach or a partner stands next to the athlete and moves a flashlight beam around on the wall.
3. The athlete follows the path of the coach's flashlight beam with her own flashlight, keeping her head still.
4. Use some smooth patterns and some quick jumps from point to point. Be sure to cover all areas of the wall and work in all regions of gaze.

Signs of Improvement

- Ability to stay right with target light while keeping head still
- Improved accuracy with increasing speed

Suggestions for Loading

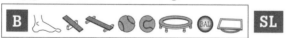

12. Four-Square Chart Fixations

Purpose   To improve these aspects of eye speed, coordination, and accuracy:

1. Left-to-right organization
2. Rhythmic flow
3. Accuracy of fixation
4. Ability to process complex figure–ground information

Materials

1. Four small letter charts (appendix I.9)
2. Metronome
3. Stopwatch

Procedure

1. Place the four letter charts on a wall in a square that is approximately eight feet by eight feet, the center of which is at eye level.
2. The athlete reads the character in the upper left corner of the upper left chart, then the character in the same position on the other charts, moving in a clockwise direction. The athlete continues across the row in the same manner and then proceeds to consecutive rows.

Add a metronome at about 40 beats per minute, and speed up to 60 beats per minute with improvement.

Signs of Improvement

Ability to perform the task at a faster metronome speed or to complete more letters in a specific time

Suggestions for Loading

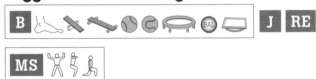

13. VDP Ball

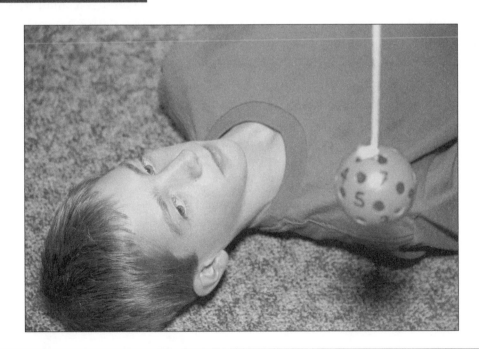

Figure 4.6 VDP ball.

Purpose   To more accurately and effortlessly control eye movements

Materials   Ball on a string with a small point to focus on (such as a small stick-on letter or number or dot drawn with a marker), swung by the coach or a partner

Procedure

1. The athlete lies flat on his back on the floor under the ball.
2. The coach or a partner swings the ball from side to side, from head to toe, and in circles while athlete follows with his eyes only, keeping his head still, focusing on the small spot on the bottom of the ball.
3. Start slowly and increase speed as the athlete's ability increases. The athlete should be sure to maintain smooth eye movements and keep his head still.
4. Progress from using both eyes simultaneously to using one eye at a time.

Signs of Improvement

*   Ability to make smooth, accurate eye movements with head held still
*   Ability to track accurately with both eyes simultaneously and with one eye at a time

Suggestions for Loading

14. VDP Ball With Thinking

Purpose   To develop the ability to maintain smooth, accurate eye movements while thinking

Materials   Ball on string with a small point to focus on (such as a small stick-on letter or dot drawn with a marker), swung by the coach or a partner

Procedure

1. The athlete lies flat on her back on the floor under the ball.
2. The coach or a partner swings the ball from side to side, from head to toe, and in circles approximately 6 to 12 inches from the athlete's face while athlete follows with her eyes only, keeping her head still, focusing on the small spot on the bottom of the ball.
3. While the athlete is tracking the ball, the coach asks her to do math problems, spell words, or solve similar problems.
4. The coach makes sure that the athlete's eye movements do not stop when answering questions and that the athlete's head remains still.

Signs of Improvement   Ability to follow the path of the swinging ball with smooth, accurate eye movements while performing the thinking tasks

Suggestions for Loading

15. Saccade Column Movements

Purpose   To develop fast and accurate saccadic movements

Materials   Saccade column chart (appendix I.10)

Procedure

1. The athlete sits or stands straight and maintains a good reading distance from the chart.
2. The athlete reads from alternating columns down the page, holding his head still, as quickly as possible.
3. The athlete tries to decrease the amount of time required to read the entire page.
4. The athlete repeats steps 1 through 3 while the coach or a partner holds the chart approximately five feet in front of athlete and moves it in a variety of directions (clockwise, counterclockwise, in a figure 8, up, down, etc.).

Signs of Improvement

- Ability to read from one column to another without losing one's place
- Ability to meet speed goals without moving one's head or losing one's place

Suggestions for Loading

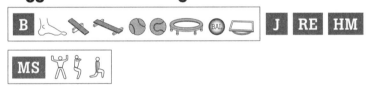

16. Slow Pursuits

Purpose   To train the eye to follow an object accurately and smoothly. This is an excellent warm-up activity not only for eye movements but also for head and cervical range of motion.

Materials   Bead string or other target

Procedure

1. The athlete holds the target directly in front of himself at normal, comfortable reading distance and slowly moves the target to the left until he can no longer fixate on the target or its image breaks in two.
2. Once the target reaches the athlete's visual limit, the athlete brings it back to center and repeats to the right, up, down, up and left, up and right, down and left, down and right.
3. Next the athlete moves his head instead of the target in the various directions. The athlete holds the target as still as possible while moving his head to the left, to the right, up, down, and so on.
4. The athlete should try to move his head in a wide, smooth motion without losing fixation or having the image of the target break in two.

5. Finally, the athlete moves his head and the target at the same time in opposite directions. For example, if the athlete moves the target to the right, he moves his head to the left at the same speed as the target. Repeat in all directions.

Signs of Improvement

- Increased range of movement without losing fixation or having image break in two
- Ability to perform movements of increasing difficulty with ease

Suggestions for Loading

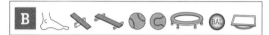

Vergence Exercises

Flexible vergence (convergence and divergence) allows the athlete to shift the distance at which the eyes are aiming quickly, easily, and accurately, as when following a softball from the bat into the outfielder's glove. The following exercises train both convergence (eyes moving inward) and divergence (eyes moving outward).

17. Near–Far Rocking

Purpose   To develop accurate focusing in each eye when looking from near to far

Materials

1. Distance letter chart (appendix I.11)
2. Two near point targets

Procedure

1. Place the distance chart across the room where it is barely readable. The athlete holds a point target in each hand at arm's length.
2. The athlete covers the left eye with the left target and looks at the near target in the right hand at arm's length.
3. The athlete slowly brings the near point target from arm's length to about six inches from the right eye, until it begins to blur.
4. The athlete then suddenly covers the right eye with the right target, uncovers the left eye, and reads three or four letters from the top row of the distance chart.
5. When the letters on the distance chart are clear, the athlete looks at the left near target now held at arm's length. Repeat steps 3 through 5 on the other side.

Variation   Vary the instructions for the distance chart. For example, read the first three letters of each line, read the first and fifth letters of each line, and so on.

Aspects to Emphasize

- Keeping both far and near targets clear and in focus
- Ability to read more letters and to keep one's place on the near and far targets

Signs of Improvement
- Increased number of letters completed in a given time
- Increased accuracy within a given time

Suggestions for Loading

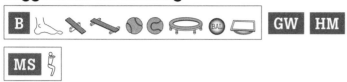

18. Opaque Lifesaver Card

Purpose   To enhance binocular vision

Materials   Opaque lifesaver card (appendix I.12) and pencil

Procedure

1. Use only the bottom set of lifesavers on the card. It may be helpful to clip a blank white paper over the others.

2. The athlete holds a pencil centered between the lower edges of the bottom circles. The athlete looks directly at the tip of the lead and observes the circles on either side without looking directly at them.

3. The athlete slowly moves the pencil toward her nose (always looking at the pencil tip and keeping it centered between the two lifesavers) until she sees four circles.

4. The athlete continues moving the pencil toward her nose and observes the inner two circles approach each other until they overlap and superimpose. She should then see three circles. The athlete should stop moving the pencil at this point.

5. The middle circle should appear smaller and closer than the original two circles.

6. Next, the athlete tries to make the letters on the circle appear clear and in focus on the middle circle by looking far away. The athlete should remember to keep her eyes crossed.

7. The athlete proceeds to the next set of lifesavers. The difficulty increases with each higher set.

8. When all these steps are mastered, the athlete can try a small, gentle "no" or "yes" head motion during the exercise. The athlete should keep her eyes on the pencil tip and keep the middle lifesaver always visible and clear. When this can be done, the athlete can try removing the pencil without moving her eyes and see if the image of the middle lifesaver can be maintained. When clarity is maintained without the pencil, the athlete can again try small, gentle head motions. The athlete can also bring the card closer to her face and then move the card away from her face while maintaining the image's clarity.

Signs of Improvement   Increased ability to recognize a central lifesaver quickly and easily and move up the chart without difficulty

Suggestions for Loading

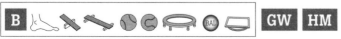

19. Hot Dog in the Sky

Purpose   To to control eye movements and flexibility of the visual system

Materials   Athlete's own index fingers

Procedure

1. The athlete extends her arms out in front, makes fists, and extends her index fingers to point at each other. The tips of the index fingers should be approximately 1/4 inch apart.

2. The athlete looks through her fingers and lets her eyes become unfocussed until she sees an illusion of a central, suspended object similar to a hot dog.

3. Once the hot dog image appears, the athlete keeps the image between the two index fingers while moving the hands in a circular motion.

4. The last modification of this exercise is to keep the image of the hot dog suspended between the two index fingers while moving the hands closer to and farther away from the face.

Signs of Improvement

1. Improved ability to maintain a single, clear and distinct hot dog image while moving the hands in a circular motion.

2. Improved ability to maintain a single, clear and distinct hot dog image while moving the fingers closer to the face and then back out again to arms' length.

3. Improved ability to maintain a single, clear and distinct hot dog image while performing a combination of the above.

Suggestions for Loading

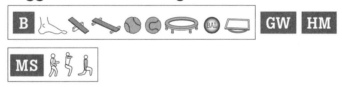

20. Pencil Push-Ups

Purpose   To help the eyes work together more accurately and efficiently for sustained periods of time

Materials

1. Pencil or pen
2. Tape measure

Procedure

Level 1

1. The athlete sits in a relaxed, balanced posture.

2. The athlete holds the pencil at arm's length straight out along her midline at nose level. The athlete should fixate on the pencil point. Make sure she can see it clearly and without double vision before she proceeds.

3. The athlete slowly moves the pencil closer to her nose, keeping her eyes on the pencil point. The athlete may need to be reminded to breathe. As she moves the pencil closer, the point may start to become blurry, and she may feel her eyes turning in. This is normal convergence.

4. It is important for the athlete to move the pencil slowly and to be aware of how it feels to look close. If one eye turns out or if athlete starts to see double, stop the pencil at that point.

5. The athlete should try to regain a single, clear view of the pencil point by turning both eyes in, aimed at the point. If she can do so, she can continue moving the pencil in as close to her nose as possible without seeing double and with both eyes turned in.

6. If the athlete is unable to regain a single view of the pencil point, she may need to move the pencil farther away. She should do this until she regains one image of the pencil point and can maintain it steadily with both eyes turned in. Once she has done this, she can again move the pencil closer, as close to her nose as possible while maintaining one pencil point and both eyes turned in.

7. Pencil push-ups are best done in short work periods several times throughout the day. The goal is to bring the pencil to the nose, or within one inch of it, consistently without the pencil image becoming double or the athlete's eyes losing alignment. The goal is to be able to repeat this five times without any visual fatigue or visual discomfort.

Level 2

1. Once the basic pencil push-ups have been mastered, near–far push-ups help build eye-teaming skill and flexibility.

2. The athlete holds a pencil at arm's length, straight ahead along the midline. Make sure he can see it clearly and without double vision before he proceeds.

3. The athlete begins moving the pencil closer to his nose, keeping both eyes aligned on the point while its image remains single. The athlete moves the pencil in a few inches, then stops, looks far away across the room, holds for a count of 4, and then looks back at the pencil. The goal is to be able to look back at the pencil and have the eyes quickly align on the point and see it without double vision. The athlete repeats this several times.

4. When this becomes easy, the athlete moves the pencil in a few inches closer each time, stopping the pencil and looking away and back for several cycles.

5. The goal is to bring the pencil to the nose, or within one inch of it, consistently, doing several cycles of "jump looking" along the way.

Signs of Improvement

• Ability to maintain clear, single vision when pushing the pencil up to the nose

• Ability to focus, look off into space, and then refocus quickly and accurately

Suggestions for Loading

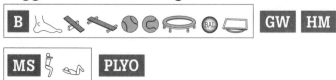

Sequencing Exercises

Sequencing helps the athlete attain and organize visual information. Sequencing helps the athlete see the greatest amount of information in the shortest amount of time. Sequencing also helps the athlete effectively attain abstract visual concepts, such as complex play diagrams.

21. Auditory Span With Vision

Purpose   To develop auditory span (i.e., the ability to recall a sequence of letters or numbers with increasing difficulty through time) for numbers using visual and visualization strategies

Materials   Written list of numbers

Procedure

1. The coach or a partner calls out three numbers in a monotone. The athlete repeats the numbers. When the athlete can do this accurately, the coach calls out four numbers. The coach increases the number sequence until the athlete misses 2 out of 10. Then the coach drops back to the previous sequence length and practices until the athlete is ready to go on to the next level.

2. The coach calls out the sequence of numbers, and the athlete repeats the numbers in the reverse order. This can be difficult. Work at the level at which the athlete can succeed.

3. Do this exercise under these three different visual conditions. Record which work best:

    a. Looking directly at the coach's face

    b. Looking at nothing in particular (e.g., at the ceiling)

    c. With eyes closed

Questions for the Athlete

- Which of the three ways was easiest? Why?
- How did your eye position change your performance of this exercise?

22. Hand Sequencing

Purpose   To improve sequential processing

Materials   Hand sequencing sheet for the coach or a partner (see appendix C)

Procedure   The coach or a partner sits opposite the athlete at a table. The coach shows the athlete a sequence of hand motions: palm down on table (P), side of hand on table (S), or fist on table (F). The athlete repeats the sequence of hand motions that the coach shows. For example, if the coach shows P, P, S (palm down, palm down, side of hand), the athlete repeats the same pattern. Levels 1 to 4 use only one hand.

Level 1   Do two motions, for example, P, P or S, P. The athlete repeats the same sequence.

Level 2   Do three motions, for example, P, S, P or F, S, P or P, P, P. The athlete repeats the same sequence.

Level 3   Do four motions, for example, P, P, F, S or P, S, S, F. The athlete repeats the same sequence.

Level 4   Do five motions, for example, P, P, S, S, F or S, F, F, P, P. The athlete repeats the same sequence.

Level 5   The coach does four motions but alternates hands, for example, right hand P, left hand F, right hand P, and left hand S. The athlete has to use the same hands in the same sequence as the coach.

Signs of Improvement   Ability to perform multiple sequences accurately

23. Picture Memories

Purpose   To improve powers of observation

Materials   Magazine pictures

Procedure   Cut out two pictures from a magazine. Mark an X on the wall, and put one picture to the left of the X and the other picture to the right of the X. The athlete stands directly in front of and looks at the X.

Level 1   The athlete looks at the picture on the left for 10 seconds. The athlete closes his eyes, counts to 10 out loud, and then, with eyes closed, describes as many details of the picture as possible from memory. Repeat with the picture on the right.

Level 2   The athlete looks at the picture on the left for 10 seconds. Then the athlete looks at the picture on the right and, while looking at that picture, describes as many details as possible of the picture on the left. Repeat with the pictures on the opposite sides.

24. Sequence Memory Skills

Purpose   To train sequence memory skills

Materials   No special equipment is required

Procedure

1. Assign letters or numbers to different objects in a room or sport equipment (such as cones, balls, or tackling dummies) on the field. For example, the sofa is A, the lamp is B, the window is C, the table is D. These assignments are verbally explained to the athlete; the objects are not physically labeled.
2. The athlete runs to the objects in sequence.
3. Vary the sequence (e.g., CBAD or ACDB), and gradually increase the length of the sequence.

4. Vary the delivery of the sequence to be carried out; present it sometimes orally and sometimes in written form.

5. The coach can also assign letters or numbers to parts of the athlete's body and ask the athlete to move those parts in sequence.

Signs of Improvement

- Ability to correctly carry out the sequence command without error or hesitation
- Ability to replicate sequences presented orally or in writing
- Ability to remember sequences of increasing length

Eye–Hand and Eye–Foot Coordination Exercises

Eye–hand and eye–foot coordination are extremely important for athletes to respond rapidly. Even sports that rely predominantly on eye–hand coordination, such as throwing and catching sports, require significant eye–foot coordination to enable the athlete to get into the best position to throw and catch. Development of eye–foot coordination improves any athlete's sport abilities.

25. Letter Tracking and Ball Bouncing

Purpose   To develop laterality and motor skill

Materials   A 20/20 eye chart (appendix I.1) and sport-appropriate ball

Procedure   The athlete slowly walks toward the eye chart placed at eye level on the wall about five feet away.

Level 1   As the athlete walks toward the chart, she calls out a letter for each step taken. The letters should be called out from left to right.

Level 2 Variations

- As the athlete walks toward the chart, he calls out the leg he is stepping on before calling out the letter, for example, "right leg" and then the letter.
- The athlete bounces a ball and then takes a step while calling out a letter. Again, the letters should be called out from left to right. The athlete alternates bouncing the ball with the right hand and then the left. The ball is bounced once for each letter.
- The athlete alternates between the right and left hands and calls out which hand is bouncing the ball before she calls out the letter.

Signs of Improvement
Increased ability to accurately read more letters in a specific time while maintaining control of the ball

Suggestions for Loading
SL

26. Straw Piercing

Purpose   To improve eye–hand coordination and peripheral vision

Materials   Drinking straw, uncooked spaghetti

Procedure

1. The coach or a partner holds a straw horizontally in front of the athlete, approximately 16 inches away from the athlete's nose, with the ends pointing to the sides.

2. The athlete holds one strand of spaghetti in each hand, approximately eight inches from each end of the straw.

3. While looking intently at the center of the straw, the athlete must attempt to pierce the two ends of the straw simultaneously, one end with each hand.

4. If the spaghetti misses the opening, the athlete should pull his hand back six inches from the straw and try again.

5. Repeat with the straw held at different heights, requiring different positions of gaze.

Suggestions for Loading

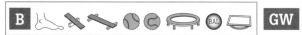

27. Spaghetti in Straw

Purpose   To develop the ability to fixate on target accurately in all regions of gaze and to improve eye–hand integration

Materials   Drinking straw, uncooked spaghetti

Procedure

1. The coach or a partner holds the straw in various positions requiring all directions of gaze, and the athlete inserts the spaghetti in the straw.

2. Be sure athlete keeps her head still and moves only her eyes to locate the straw.

3. The athlete should use both right and left hands to insert the spaghetti.

Signs of Improvement   Ability to locate straw and accurately insert spaghetti without head movement

Suggestions for Loading

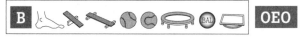

28. Punching O's

Purpose   To improve eye–hand coordination. This is an excellent group activity to enhance team building, eye–hand coordination, and binocular vision.

Materials

1. Toothpick
2. Punching O's exercise chart (appendix I.13)
3. Styrofoam® block, approximately 8 1/2 by 11 inches

Procedure

1. Place the O chart on top of the Styrofoam block.
2. The athlete punches the center of the O's with a toothpick for 60 seconds. Determine the number of O's that were pierced in their centers, within their boundaries.

Signs of Improvement   Increased speed and accuracy in a given time period

Suggestions for Loading

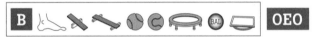

29. Penny Drop

Purpose

1. To develop accurate eye–hand coordination
2. To enhance efficiency of specific muscle movements
3. To enhance skill in predicting location in space
4. To integrate visual and auditory information
5. To enhance pursuit movements

Materials

1. Containers such as cups of various sizes
2. A penny or other small object (e.g., bead, button)
3. A clicker or small bell (optional)

Procedure

1. The athlete holds the penny lightly between the thumb and forefinger of his preferred hand. The coach or a partner stands facing the athlete, holding a small container with one hand. With the other hand, the coach holds a clicker or bell out of the athlete's sight.
2. The coach moves the container continuously in all directions within reach of the athlete.
3. The athlete keeps the penny directly above the container as it moves around. The athlete tracks the container visually and with his own hand while keeping his head still at all times.

4. When the coach clicks the clicker or gives a verbal cue, the athlete must release the penny immediately. If the athlete has been accurately tracking the moving container, the penny falls directly into the container.

5. Continue the activity until the athlete has five consecutive hits. The athlete may alternate hands after each consecutive hit.

Variations

• As the athlete's skill increases, use progressively smaller containers.

• Have the athlete perform the activity while solving math problems given by the coach.

Signs of Improvement

• Athlete successfully drops the penny into the container on five of five tries.

• Athlete performs accurately using containers of various sizes.

• Athlete releases the penny immediately at the sound of the clicker.

• Athlete does not move head.

• Athlete performs accurately while doing loading activities or cognitive tasks, such as math problems or naming state capitals.

Suggestions for Loading

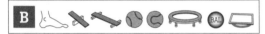

30. Decode Chart

Purpose

1. To develop eye–hand coordination
2. To reinforce tracking skills and right–left awareness
3. To improve ability to follow sequential directions

Materials

1. Decode chart (appendix I.14)
2. Sport-appropriate ball

Procedure

1. The coach or a partner holds the chart in front of the athlete or hangs the chart on the wall at eye level.

2. Each figure on the chart represents a different task for the athlete to do. These are examples:

Circle: Bounce ball with left hand.

Square: Bounce ball with right hand.

Triangle: Bounce ball with both hands.

Rectangle: Throw ball in the air and catch it.

3. Reading from left to right across each row, the athlete performs the appropriate actions.

4. Vary the actions to be performed.

Signs of Improvement   Ability to perform correct action in sequence without error or hesitation

Comment   This is an excellent team or group activity.

31. Continuous Motion

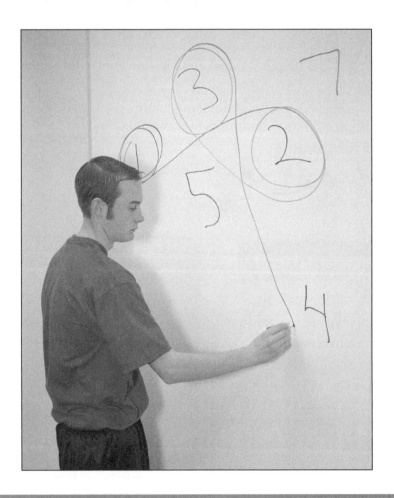

Figure 4.7   Continuous motion.

Purpose   To develop rhythmic, accurate eye–hand movement and a wide field of vision

Materials   Chalkboard and chalk or paper and pencil, stopwatch for timing the exercise

Procedure

1. The coach or a partner writes the numbers 1 through 20 in random order on a three- to four-foot area of the chalkboard, leaving several inches of space around each number.
2. The athlete takes the chalk in her preferred hand and, starting at number 1, circles each number in order once in a counterclockwise direction.
3. Without stopping or removing the chalk from the board, the number 2 is located and circled in the same manner.
4. The athlete continues circling numbers in sequence up through the number 10.
5. When moving the chalk from one number to the next, the athlete must avoid touching or crossing any number. The athlete must keep the chalk moving during the search for the next number to be circled.
6. The athlete uses her nonpreferred hand to repeat the procedure for numbers 11 through 20, this time circling each number three times in a clockwise direction.
7. When the athlete can perform efficiently at the chalkboard, repeat the procedure on paper with pencil.
8. After athlete becomes proficient at the exercise, the coach times the trials with the stopwatch, looking for improvement with each successive trial.

Aspects to Emphasize

- Smooth, continuous control of the chalk and avoid contact with numbers
- Increased speed and accuracy in the visual search for the next number

Signs of Improvement

Increased speed and accuracy with both dominant and nondominant hands

Suggestions for Loading

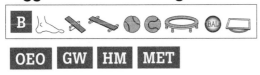

32. Catcho

Purpose   To improve the ability to identify right and left in relationship to self and in space

Materials   Beanbag

Procedure

1. The coach or a partner and the athlete toss the beanbag back and forth to each other. The coach calls out which hand the athlete is to use to catch the beanbag.
2. As the athlete improves the ability to catch with the correct hand, toss the beanbag back and forth faster.

3. Add an extra beanbag. As the athlete throws one beanbag to the coach, the coach simultaneously throws the other beanbag back to the athlete. The coach calls out which hand the athlete is to use to catch the second beanbag.

4. To make this exercise more difficult, have the athlete turn his back to the coach. The coach throws the beanbag over the athlete's shoulder while calling out which hand to catch the beanbag with. The coach can either throw the beanbag over the same shoulder as the catching hand or over the opposite shoulder to make the exercise more difficult.

Suggestions for Loading

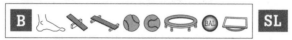

33. Slap Jack

Purpose   To develop form constancy, internal detail, speed of recognition, eye–hand coordination, and fine motor control; to promote rapid and accurate visual recognition of the designated "slap" card without any false slaps to similar cards. This is a great team-building activity that can be played while traveling to a competition or while waiting before the start of the contest.

Materials   Deck of playing cards

Procedure

1. Two players sit across from each other at a table or on the floor.

2. Shuffle the cards and divide them equally between the two players, keeping the cards face down and directly in front of each player.

3. Each player alternately turns over the top card on her stack and places it face up in a single stack between the two players.

4. When a jack is turned up, each player tries to slap it with the hand she is not using to turn over the cards.

5. The player who slaps the jack first gets the face-up pile of cards in the middle and adds it to the bottom of her stack. If there is a question as to which player was first, the player whose hand is on the bottom takes the pile.

6. The game continues until one player obtains all the cards and is then pronounced the winner. The game also may be played with a time limit. After the allotted time, the player with the most cards is the winner.

Variations   Any other card or cards can be selected as the card to slap, further challenging the athletes' form constancy and visual recognition skills.

34. Bimanual Circles

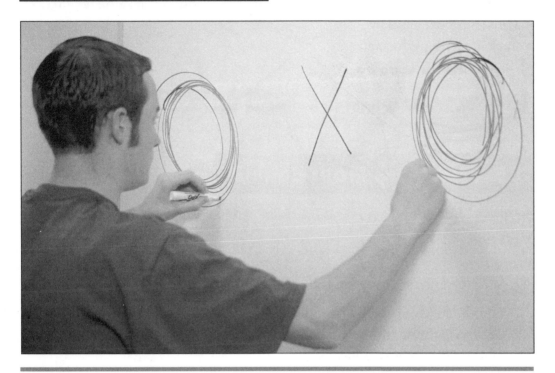

Figure 4.8   Bimanual circles.

Purpose

1. To improve visual motor skills
2. To improve bimanual integration, or ambidextrous abilities
3. To improve laterality and directionality

Materials   Whiteboard or chalkboard and appropriate writing implement

Procedure

1. The athlete stands in front of the board with a piece of chalk or marker in each hand.
2. The athlete makes an X at a level slightly lower than eye level.
3. The coach tells the athlete, "Keep your eyes on the X."
4. The athlete draws two circles about the diameter of a basketball, one with each hand. The circle with the left hand is made with a clockwise motion, and the circle with the right hand is made with a counterclockwise motion. The circles should be equally round, equal in size, equally far from the X, and both at the same height.
5. The athlete should start the circles at the top and go around six times at a rate of a circle a second, counting each time the chalk passes the top of the circles.
6. The coach should not interrupt these circles. When the athlete is finished, the coach asks him to step back and look at the circles. They will probably not look very good, but the coach should say, "Okay, you followed the directions very well. What do you think? Did your hands work equally well?" The answer is likely to be an excuse regarding the athlete's handedness.

Signs of Improvement
- Circles are drawn an equal distance from the X and at the same height.
- Circles appear similar.
- Task is easily performed.

Suggestions for Loading

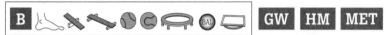

35. Beanbags From Behind

Purpose   To improve visualization, reaction time, and peripheral awareness

Materials   Beanbag

Procedure

Level 1
1. The athlete stands with her back to the coach or a partner.
2. The coach throws the beanbag while calling out "left side" or "right side."
3. The athlete catches the beanbag.

Level 2   Follow the preceding instructions without stating on what side beanbag will be thrown.

Signs of Improvement   Ability to catch the beanbag easily and smoothly

Suggestions for Loading

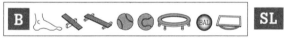

36. Juggling

Purpose   To improve eye–hand coordination

Materials   Three equally weighted objects (e.g., beanbags, tennis balls, baseballs). In general, the lighter the object, the easier it is to juggle.

Procedure
1. There are many ways to learn to juggle, for example, from a video, over the Internet, or from a friend.
2. The athlete may find it easiest to start with two objects.
3. The key to success in juggling is practice, practice, practice!

Signs of Improvement

- Ability to juggle with a sport-specific object or implement (But use hockey pucks rather than hockey sticks!)
- Ability to juggle three or more objects
- Ability to juggle three or more different objects

Suggestions for Loading

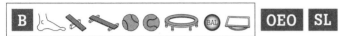

37. Broomstick Balancing

Purpose   To develop fine motor control

Materials   Broomstick, wand, dowel, racket, or other sport-specific implement

Procedure

1. The athlete places the end of the broomstick or implement in the palm of the hand.
2. The athlete learns to balance the stick while standing.
3. Once the athlete becomes proficient with one hand, she switches hands and learns to balance with the other.
4. Next the athlete learns to balance the stick on the index finger.
5. Then the athlete tries to move the stick from fingertip to fingertip without dropping it.
6. Repeat steps 4 and 5 with the opposite hand.

Signs of Improvement   Increased ability to balance broomstick while simultaneously performing balance loading exercises

Suggestions for Loading

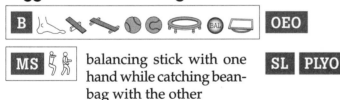

balancing stick with one hand while catching beanbag with the other

38. Egg Carton Catch

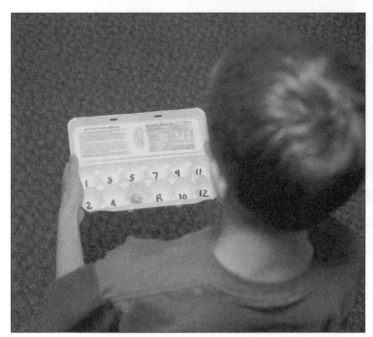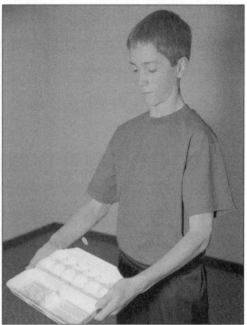

Figure 4.9 Egg carton catch.

Purpose   To improve fine motor control, eye–hand coordination, and eye movement speed and accuracy

Materials

1. A 12- or 18-egg carton
2. A quarter
3. Marking pen
4. Stopwatch or timer

Procedure

1. Number the inside of each egg compartment in the carton sequentially, starting with number 1 in the upper left compartment, 2 in the compartment below that (the lower left), up to 12 (or 18) in the lower right corner.

2. Place the quarter in cup 1.

3. The coach or a partner says "go" and starts the stopwatch, and the athlete tries to flip the quarter up out of cup 1 into cup 2, then from cup 2 to cup 3, and so on. The goal is to flip the quarter from one cup to the next in sequence in the least amount of time.

4. Once the athlete becomes proficient at the basic task, try the following variations:

   a. The athlete flips the quarter across one row of cups and back the other, in this order: 1, 3, 5, 7, 9, 11, 12, 10, 8, 6, 4, 2.

   b. The coach calls out a random number to which the athlete must flip the coin as quickly as possible.

   c. The coach calls out simple math problems, such as "3 + 6," and the athlete must solve the problem and get quarter to land in the cup that corresponds to the answer.

Signs of Improvement   Increased speed and accuracy

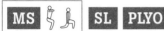 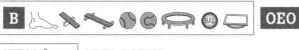

39. Flip Sticks

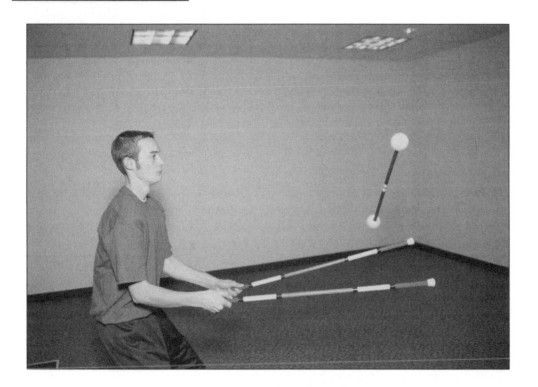

Figure 4.10   Flip sticks.

Purpose   To develop eye–hand coordination and eye movement speed and accuracy

Materials

1. Two dowels approximately three feet long by three fourths of an inch in diameter (catching sticks)

2. One dowel approximately two feet long by three eighths of an inch in diameter (flip stick)

3. Two 3/4-inch rubber end caps and two old tennis balls

4. Colored electrical tape, preferably in these six colors: red, blue, green, yellow, black, and white

Procedure

1. Wrap one-half inch of white tape on one end of each of the two longer dowels (catching sticks). Then wrap nine inches of blue tape, followed by one-half inch

of white tape, then nine inches of red tape, one-half inch of white tape, nine inches of yellow tape, one-half inch of white tape, nine inches of green tape, and one-half inch of white tape on the end of the dowel. Make sure each of the long dowels looks the same. Place an end cap on one end of each dowel.

2. Wrap black tape around the entire length of the shorter dowel (flip stick), and then place a tennis ball on each end.

3. The athlete holds the green end of a catching stick in each hand and places the flip stick on the blue end. Now, using fine motor movements, the athlete tosses and rotates the flip stick one-half turn clockwise and then catches it on the two catching sticks. Then the athlete tosses the flip stick one-half turn counterclockwise and again catches it on the catch sticks. If the flip stick falls on the floor, the athlete picks it up and tries again.

4. After mastering this technique, the athlete can try the following:

   a. Repeat step 3, but toss the flip stick from the blue portion of the stick and catch it on the red portion. Then toss it from the red portion and catch it on the yellow portion. Finally, toss it from the yellow portion and catch it on the green portion.

   b. Repeat steps 3 and 4a with a full rotation of the flip stick.

   c. Toss the flip stick half a turn and catch it with eyes closed.

   d. The coach or a partner calls out a color while the flip stick is in the air, and the athlete tries to catch the flip stick on the portion of that color.

   e. The flip stick must land in the colored areas, not on the white line, for a flip to count.

   f. Within minutes, most athletes will come up with endless other variations of flip-stick catching.

Signs of Improvement   Increased speed, accuracy, and complexity of tasks without dropping flip stick

Suggestions for Loading

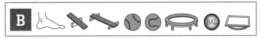

   playing catch with a partner using
another pair of catching sticks

Visualization Exercises

Visualization is the ability to picture an object or situation in the mind's eye. This key component of athletic skill is necessary for consistent performance and concentration.

40. Delayed Memory

Purpose   To improve visual memory

Materials   Deck of playing cards

Procedure

1. The athlete sits comfortably with good posture at a desk or table. The coach or a partner reads these instructions to the athlete: "I am going to show you two cards, one at a time. Then I am going to ask you what the first one was. Then I will show you a third card and ask you what the second one was, and so on. Each time you will be asked to remember the card you saw *before* the one you saw last."

2. The coach shows the athlete one card and places it face down. Then the coach shows the athlete another card and places it face down. The coach points to the first card and asks the athlete to identify it.

3. The coach shows the athlete a third card and places it face down. The coach points to the second card and asks the athlete to identify it.

4. This procedure continues until all 52 cards have been used.

5. The cards that the athlete identifies correctly are put in one stack, and the errors in another stack.

6. As the athlete's performance improves, the number of cards shown before the athlete is asked to identify the first card may be increased.

Aspects to Emphasize

- Good posture and working distance
- Awareness of the rest of the room

Signs of Improvement

- Accurately identifying a greater number of cards
- Less time necessary for each identification
- Increased number of cards between the card shown and the one identified

Suggestion for Loading

MET

41. Space Matching

Purpose

1. To improve sense of location in relation to surroundings
2. To visualize distance using some form of measurement

Materials   Length of string

Procedure

1. The athlete estimates the number of steps it will take to walk to some object across the room or across the field. The athlete then paces the distance off to check the estimate.

2. The athlete estimates the number of steps it will take to travel half or other fractions of the distance to an object.

3. The athlete estimates the number of steps between two objects and paces it off.

4. The athlete estimates the number of steps to travel half or other fractions of the distance between two objects across the room or across the field.

5. The athlete estimates the width, height, and depth of objects and holds just enough string between his hands that he estimates would fit around the object. The athlete checks the string against the real object. If the original estimate is inaccurate, the athlete holds the correct length of string and returns to the original location to look again at the object while feeling the actual size represented by the string.

Signs of Improvement

- Ability to accurately judge the number of steps between self and object
- Ability to accurately judge the number of steps between objects at a distance
- Ability to accurately estimate with the hands the width, height, and depth of objects at a distance
- Ability to make fractional estimates

42. Quick Exposure

Purpose

1. To increase the capacity and efficiency of the visual memory
2. To increase peripheral awareness

Materials   Stack of three-by-five-inch cards. Every other card has a number or series of numbers on it.

Procedure

1. The athlete sits with good posture in a room or an area with good lighting.
2. The athlete holds the cards tightly at one end with the nondominant hand.
3. The athlete flips the cards with thumb of the dominant hand so as to expose a numbered card and then without delay flips to the next blank card and stops.
4. The athlete closes her eyes and repeats out loud the number or number sequence presented on the card.
5. The athlete or a partner checks the answer.
6. Repeat.

Variations

- Mix numbers with letters.
- Decrease the size of the numbers or letters or increase length of the sequences.
- Make cards showing plays, formations, or other sport-relevant visual information.

Signs of Improvement

- Ability to repeat contents of cards with increasing accuracy
- Ability to repeat contents of cards with decreasing exposure times
- Ability to accurately repeat sequences of increasing length or complexity

43. Parquetry Patterns

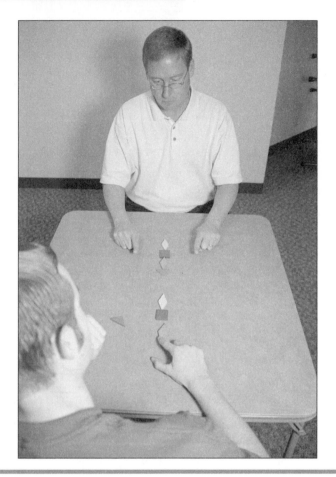

Figure 4.11   Parquetry patterns.

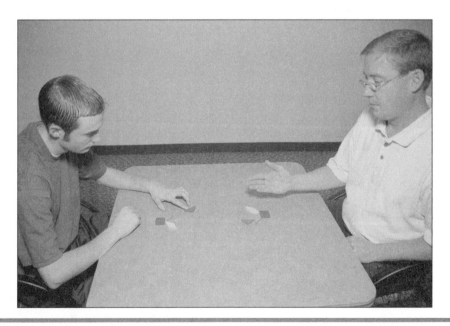

Figure 4.12   Parquetry pattern exercise.

Purpose

1. To develop ability to visualize the parts necessary to form a whole
2. To be able to visually manipulate objects in space

Materials   Parquetry blocks. See appendix E for instructions for making your own.

Procedure

1. The coach or a partner puts the parquetry blocks together into a pattern, and then the athlete uses the other set of blocks to construct the same design next to it.
2. The coach then moves to the opposite side of the table and faces the athlete. The coach instructs the athlete to replicate the design as if the coach were to slide the pattern toward the athlete without actually sliding the design toward the athlete. The coach uses the instruction, "Pretend that I am sliding this pattern toward you. Reproduce the pattern exactly as you saw it before I slid it toward you."
3. The athlete then visualizes the coach's pattern as if it were flipped over with a spatula toward the athlete and reproduces the visualized pattern.
4. In another variation, the coach asks the athlete to replicate the pattern as if the pattern were rotated clockwise 90, 180, or 270 degrees, and then to replicate it rotated counterclockwise.
5. Begin with less complicated patterns and proceed to more difficult ones.
6. The coach lets the athlete study the pattern and then places an opaque piece of paper over the pattern so that the athlete can no longer actually see the pattern to replicate. The athlete must visualize the pattern and orientation of the pieces in the mind's eye.

Signs of Improvement

- Ability to quickly and accurately reproduce complex designs
- Ability to manipulate objects in the mind's eye quickly and accurately

44. Coding at the Chalkboard

Purpose   To develop young athletes' visual associations with tactile and auditory information processing

Materials   Chalkboard and whistle or buzzer

Procedure

1. The athlete stands facing chalkboard, and the coach or a partner stands behind the athlete.
2. The coach uses the whistle or buzzer to make intermittent short and long sounds. The athlete draws corresponding short and long lines on chalkboard. The athlete needs to be aware of the duration of the sound and relate it to the length of the line.
3. Repeat using a sequence of two, three, or four sounds at a time for the athlete to indicate with lines at the chalkboard.
4. The athlete decodes a series of dots and dashes drawn on the chalkboard into sounds using the buzzer or whistle.

Signs of Improvement   Ability to accurately match sound durations and line lengths

Suggestions for Loading

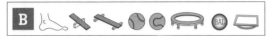

45. Ace to King

Purpose

1. To improve the ability to concentrate and attend for longer periods of time
2. To develop the ability to visualize and recall sequential arrangements

Materials   Deck of playing cards

Procedure

1. The athlete sits comfortably with good posture at a desk or table.
2. The coach or a partner sorts the deck of cards by suit; use a set of 13 cards of the same suit, from ace to king.
3. The coach shuffles the 13 cards and places them face down in a row in front of the athlete.
4. The athlete turns each card over one at a time to see which card it is and then turns it back face down.
5. Now the athlete turns the cards face up again in order, from ace to king. If a card is turned out of sequence, the athlete must turn all cards face down again and start over.
6. This task can be made easier by using only ace to six or more difficult by using two suits.

Aspects to Emphasize

- Good posture and working distance
- Awareness of entire table surface and the rest of the room

Signs of Improvement

- Ability to visualize the card sequence quickly and accurately
- Ability to increase number of cards used
- Ability to maintain awareness of other objects in room

46. Sport-Specific Visualization

Purpose   To visualize a sport-specific activity, such as slalom skiing, soccer penalty kicks, free-throw shooting, golfing

Materials

1. Sport-specific visualization sheet (appendixes I.15 through I.22) or chalkboard
2. Pencil, pen, or chalk

Procedure

1. The athlete places a pencil, pen, or chalk at the designated starting area of the drawing for the activity to be visualized.
2. The athlete visually memorizes the path of the activity or the path of the ball visualized.
3. Next the athlete closes her eyes, visualizes the activity, and draws a line from the starting point to the finish.

See the following instructions for scoring and progression of difficulty for each sport activity.

- Baseball pitcher: The pitcher "stands" on the mound with a pen and then visualizes the strike zone. The athlete then closes his eyes and traces the path of a thrown strike into the catcher's glove. Keep score of balls and strikes.

- Basketball: The player visualizes shooting free throws, three-point shots, and other shots by visualizing the court and the basket and then closing her eyes and tracing the path of the ball to the basket.

- Football: Three players, a quarterback, a wide receiver, and a defensive back, line up their pens in their respective positions on the field. First, the quarterback visualizes where he wants to throw the ball, then closes his eyes, and "passes" the ball to that point with a pen. The wide receiver sees where the quarterback passes the ball, then closes his eyes, and tries to "run" to that point with his pen. Last, the defensive back lines up, visualizes the best point to make an interception, closes his eyes, and then "runs" with his pen to that point. Play continues until a touchdown or an interception is made (it is helpful to use real plays in this visualization exercise). Placekickers and punters can also use this exercise by trying to "kick the ball" with their pens through the uprights, or punters can try to place the ball inside the 10-yard line.

- Golf: Each player uses a different colored pen. Before a golfer is ready to "swing," she visualizes the hole, places the pen on "tee box," closes her eyes, and traces the path of the ball to get to as close to the hole as possible. Once the golfer opens her eyes, one shot is completed. If a player goes out of bounds, she needs to go back to the original spot and count a stroke. If the player goes into a hazard, she has to play from the hazard. Players alternate shots until one player's pen stops in the hole.

- Skiing: Each racer uses a different colored pen. Before going through the course, each racer visualizes the gate pattern and then places the pen at the starting gate. On the command "go," the racer closes his eyes and starts drawing the path through the gates. The racer does not open his eyes until he has completed the course. One point is scored for each gate that the racer successfully completes in the correct direction. A variation is timing the race as well as scoring the number of successfully completed gates.

- Soccer: Penalty kicks, free kicks, and corner kicks can be visualized. The player places a pen on the penalty spot and visualizes the goal. The player closes her eyes and "shoots," trying to move the pen into the net. Free kicks and corner kicks can also be practiced. After visualizing the wall in relation to the goal, the player then closes her eyes and "shoots" around the wall and into a corner of the goal.

- Tennis: A player can practice serving by "standing" on the baseline, visualizing the court, close his eyes, and trying to trace the path of the serve to a predetermined spot on the opponent's side. A second player using a different colored pen "returns the serve" by trying to trace the path of the ball into a selected area on the court with eyes closed. Play continues until the ball goes out of bounds or into the net.

- Volleyball: Players practice serving by visualizing the court, closing their eyes, and then "hitting" the ball by moving the pen to a predetermined area of the court.

Suggestions for Loading

1. Two or more athletes compete.

2. Establish a consequence for athletes who lose the competition or a reward for athletes who win.

Directionality Exercises

Directionality is the ability to quickly and accurately perceive left and right and to project left and right out into space. This seemingly simple skill can become very difficult under even the simplest loading situations. By concentrating and working on developing better directionality, an athlete will find that simple left and right decisions can be made more efficiently and quickly under the stress of competition. Athletes who are aware of left and right become increasingly aware of their own bodies. Improving athletes' directionality abilities also improves their balance and field awareness.

47. VDP Charts

Purpose   To increase accuracy and coordination of eye–hand and eye–foot integration

Materials

1. VDP charts (appendixes I.23 through I.26)

2. Metronome

Procedure

Level 1

1. On the first chart (appendix I.23), the athlete calls out which side of the line the star is on: right, left, or middle. Start with the metronome at a slow speed and gradually increase the pace.

2. After this is mastered, the athlete taps the right hand to indicate that the star is to the right of the line, taps the left hand to indicate that the star is to the left, and taps both hands together if the star is in the middle.

Level 2   This exercise concentrates on the feet. The athlete follows the preceding instructions but uses the second chart (appendix I.24), in which the square represents the feet. The athlete should work slow and accurately.

Level 3   This exercise combines movement of the hands and feet. The athlete follows the same instructions but this time uses the chart in appendix I.25 and taps one foot (square) or one hand (star) at a time.

Level 4   This level combines eye, hand, and foot coordination. The athlete follows the same instructions but this time uses the chart in appendix I.26 which may require simultaneous taps of a foot (square) and a hand (star).

Signs of Improvement   Increase in the speed of the metronome with consistent, appropriate, error-free coordinating motor responses

48. Simon Says

Purpose   To improve coordination while listening to instructions

Materials   None

Procedure

1. The coach or a partner gives instructions such as "Simon says, Raise your left arm. Tap your right foot."

2. As the athlete becomes proficient at following single commands, make the task more difficult by giving commands that involve two body parts, such as "Simon says, With your right hand, touch your left ear. With your left hand, touch your right elbow."

3. As the athlete becomes more proficient, make the task more difficult by giving commands that involve three body parts, for example, "Simon says, With your right hand, touch your left knee and then your right knee. With your left hand, touch your right ear and then your right knee."

4. The important aspect of this exercise is using the right and left sides of the body in every command.

5. The following list is an example Simon Says game. These are just suggestions; the combinations are limitless.

Simon says:

1. Put your left hand on your right toe.
2. Clap your hands twice.
3. Put your left hand on your left toe.
4. Put your elbows together.
5. Touch your heels.
6. Touch your eyes.
7. Put your feet apart.
8. Touch one elbow.
9. Touch two elbows.
10. Draw a square in the air.
11. Clap one time.
12. Clasp your hands behind your neck.
13. Touch one shoulder.
14. Put your knees together.
15. Touch your right knee with your left hand.
16. Touch your left knee with your right hand.
17. Place your palms together.
18. Clap your hands twice.
19. Touch one knee and one foot.
20. Put your hands on your head.
21. Touch your nose.
22. Touch your toes with your arms crossed.

23. Touch your nose with one hand and your knee with the other.
24. Put your right hand on your left knee.
25. Cross your arms in front of your chest.
26. Put your right hand over your left eye.
27. Cross your arms in front of your chest.
28. Put your left hand on your right knee.
29. Cross your arms in front of your chest.
30. Put your right hand on your left hip.
31. Cross your arms in front of your chest.
32. Put your left hand on your right hip.
33. Cross your arms in front of your chest.
34. Put your left hand on your right foot.
35. Cross your arms in front of your chest.
36. Put your right hand on your left foot.
37. Cross your arms in front of your chest.
38. Put your left hand on your right ear.
39. Cross your arms in front of your chest.
40. Put your right hand on your left ear.
41. Cross your arms in front of your chest.
42. Put both hands on top of your head.

Signs of Improvement
Improved accuracy with time

49. Ferris Wheel

Purpose   To visualize and reproduce forms in rotated positions

Materials   Ferris wheel (appendix I.27) and pencil

Procedure
1. The coach or a partner draws a letter, number, or simple geometric shape in the top box of the form.
2. The athlete visualizes what the letter, number, or shape will look like when the form is rotated a quarter turn, a half turn, and a three-quarters turn.
3. The athlete draws the form in those rotated positions.

Note: Right triangles and irregular shapes are more difficult to visually rotate in this activity.

Signs of Improvement
- Ability to visualize the rotated forms without turning the head, body, or paper and without relying on external cues
- Ability to draw rotated forms accurately

50. Arrow Chart

Purpose   To identify directions (up, down, right, and left) quickly and confidently

Materials
1. Arrow chart (appendix I.28)
2. Metronome

Procedure

1. Attach the chart to a wall. As the coach or a partner points to each arrow, the athlete calls out the direction in which the arrow is pointing and at the same time points in that the direction.
2. Add the metronome, starting slowly and gradually increasing speed.
3. Have the athlete both call and point in the direction opposite that indicated by the arrow.
4. Have the athlete point and call in a direction that is a quarter turn clockwise or counterclockwise from that indicated by the arrow.

Signs of Improvement

- Ability to visually keep place on chart
- Ability to call directions accurately in a steady rhythm

Suggestions for Loading

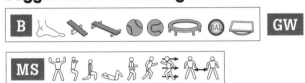

Chapter **5**

Sport-Specific *SportsVision* Training Exercises

Since the 1980s, coaches in almost every sport have come to recognize the value of sport-specific training. They have learned that with limited training time, it only makes sense to train the way you play. In the 1990s, coaches came to realize that sport-specific resistance training, year-round conditioning, and periodization are necessary for athletes to perform at the highest level. It is our sincere hope that in the 2000s, coaches in all sports will learn that *SportsVision* training and enhancement can be as effective for their athletes as other changes in the sport training model have been. But as with these other advances, *SportsVision* training has to be sport specific. In this chapter, we outline the visual motor training exercises from chapter 4 that are most beneficial for each of the sports discussed. In addition, we describe how to modify the exercises specifically for the visual demands of each sport. Finally, where appropriate, we provide suggestions for on-field or on-court *SportsVision* training for the entire team.

Table 5.1 presents the visual demands of 17 different sports. Certain positions in certain sports may have slightly different visual demands, such as ball handlers versus linemen in football; fielders, hitters, and pitchers in baseball; and goalkeepers versus field players in hockey and soccer. Certain related sports may also have slightly different visual demands, such as field versus ice hockey and the various racket sports (tennis, racquetball, squash, badminton).

SportsVision Training Progression: 30 Days to Better Sports Vision

Just as with any exercise training, a *SportsVision* training program must appropriately set the exercise variables of frequency, intensity, duration, and type of activity to achieve the optimal training benefits. However, one of the main differences between a traditional resistance training program and a *SportsVision* training program is that the athlete's eye muscles usually are already as strong as they need to be. With *SportsVision* training, the

83

Table 5.1

Visual Demands of 17 Different Sports

	Focusing	Tracking	Vergence	Sequencing	Coordination	Visualization	Directionality
Baseball	5	5	5	2	5	3	2
Basketball	4	5	5	2	5	4	3
Boxing	3	5	4	1	5	2	1
Cricket	5	5	5	2	5	3	2
Cycling	2	5	2	4	2	5	1
Diving	3	4	1	5	3	5	4
Downhill Skiing	3	5	2	4	5	5	5
Figure Skating	3	4	4	5	5	5	5
Football	4	5	5	5	5	4	4
Golf	3	3	3	5	5	5	5
Gymnastics	4	5	5	5	5	5	5
Hockey	5	5	5	3	5	2	2
Lacrosse	4	5	4	3	5	2	2
Racket Sports	5	5	5	3	5	4	3
Rugby	4	5	5	5	5	4	4
Soccer	5	5	3	4	5	4	5
Volleyball	4	5	5	2	5	3	1

Scoring: 1 = not important to 5 = very important

Adapted from Dr. Alan Sherman, with permission (1990).

goal is to increase the coordination, speed of eye movement, and conditioning of the visual system. It is important that athletes progress through the exercise program in an organized manner and try to perfect each skill or exercise to the best of their abilities. Some athletes inherently perform given skills better, and these athletes may progress through an exercise series faster than recommended. In all the years that we have been training athletes, we have *never* found an athlete in any sport who could not, through practice, improve the performance of any given visual skill. In fact, we have challenged some very elite athletes to improve their skills and been amazed at their level of improvement after training.

In our six-week training program, we ask athletes to commit to a minimum of 3 to 5 minutes for each exercise for a total of 18 to 30 minutes of training per day, five days a week, for the entire training period of six weeks. We have found that the 3- to 5-minute training period for each exercise allows significant improvement in visual skills with minimal encroachment on the athlete's valuable and limited time. However, if an athlete would like to commit more time to *SportsVision* training, there is no harm done in doing so, and in fact, the old adage "More is better" truly applies here. Resistance training has a physiologic limit to the amount, intensity, and frequency that yields optimal results. But additional *SportsVision* training time and frequency allows any athlete to maximize the results.

For each specific sport, we outline a six-week training program consisting of six different exercises. In the initial week of training, athletes should spend their time trying to perfect the basic exercise. In weeks 2 to 6, each exercise is loaded with an additional task to progressively challenge the visual system in a calculated manner. Don't be tempted to jump from the exercise in week 2 to the one in week 6; this defeats the calculated progression of each exercise and will result in frustration. For each sport, the program has been carefully planned to address the specific visual needs of that sport. However, coaches should identify players' specific weaknesses and provide additional customized training to turn that weakness into strength. This can be accomplished by assigning additional exercises and appropriate loading tasks to the exercises in a systematic progression based on the results of the pretraining evaluation. The more coaches practice *SportsVision* training with their athletes, the better they will become at customizing the training program for each athlete's needs and shortfalls.

The loading tasks increase the intensity of *SportsVision* training exercises (see the icon key on page vi). The intensity of exercises increases each week. Each week, a loading activity is added that makes an exercise significantly more difficult. (Athletes should not progress until they have mastered the previous week's activity.) Although athletes may become frustrated at the start of a new loading exercise, with practice, they will develop and enhance their visual abilities. The purpose of loading is to create a much more challenging environment for the visual and motor systems than occurs in competition. The loading activities prepare athletes for any circumstance that might occur during the game, and thus, in actual competition, the capabilities of their visual systems far exceed the demands of the game.

For each of the 17 sports that follow, we provide six sport-specific *SportsVision* training exercises. After the initial week of training, loading tasks are added to make that exercise more challenging and more fun!

Baseball and Softball

You can't hit (or catch) what you can't see. *SportsVision* can have a significant effect in sports such as baseball and softball that use small, high-velocity projectiles. These sports require tremendous binocular vision, which is a skill that can be trained. Baseball and softball players need optimal visual correction to maximize their visual performance. *SportsVision* training can improve the hitting and fielding skills of baseball and softball players of all ages and abilities. Table 5.2 outlines a *SportsVision* program for baseball and softball players.

Modifications for Baseball or Softball

1. Exercise 1, Focusing Pursuits (page 39), modified for baseball or softball by using a baseball or softball marked with five different numbers and five different letters. Each number or letter should be approximately half an inch high.

2. Exercise 2, Near–Far Eye Jumps (page 39), modified for baseball or softball by using the same ball as in exercise 1 for the near target.

3. Exercise 7, Ball Batting (page 43).

4. Exercise 9, Bead String (page 46), modified for baseball or softball by making the string the distance from the pitcher's mound to home plate (60 feet, 6 inches long for baseball; 43 to 50 feet for softball).

5. Exercise 26, Straw Piercing (page 59).

6. Exercise 35, Beanbags From Behind (page 66), modified for baseball or softball by using a regulation baseball or softball and glove.

Table 5.2

Baseball and Softball SportsVision Training Program

		Week 1	Week 2	Week 3	Week 4	Week 5	Week 6
Focusing	Exercise 1	B (foot)	B (pencil)	RE	B (foot) GW	MS (figures)
Focusing	Exercise 2	B (board)	RE	B (balls)	HM	B (BAL)
Tracking	Exercise 7	MET	B (pencil) RE	B (foot) MET	SL	B (trampoline) MET SL
Tracking	Exercise 9	GW	HM	B (balls)	B (BAL)	B (foot) HM
Coordination	Exercise 26	GW	B (pencil) GW	B (pencil)	B (board)	B (BAL)
Coordination	Exercise 35	B (trampoline)	B (balls)	SL	B (trampoline) SL	B (balls) SL

7. Group activity (can be done by small group or entire team): Exercise 47, VDP Charts (page 78). Perform this at the end of each training session in weeks 1 to 6.

8. *SportsVision* field training:

   a. Color seams of baseball or softball for use in batting practice or during catch.

   b. Put numbers or letters on a ball when playing catch. See how many letters athletes can see before catching the ball.

   c. Play waffle ball, hitting and fielding, under a strobe light.

   d. Play catch with a waffle or tennis ball under a strobe light. Practice throwing balls in the air, and practice catching ground balls.

Basketball

The no-look pass in basketball epitomizes the application of *SportsVision*. A guard who runs down the floor and looks one way, but passes the ball in the other direction requires eye–hand coordination, balance, near–far focusing, tracking of his teammates and the opponents, peripheral awareness, and visualization to make the play. Shooting skills and proficiency can also be increased with *SportsVision* training. The player needs to accurately judge his distance from the rim as well as where the defenders are or may be coming from. He needs to develop eye–hand and even eye–body coordination to perfect his touch and technical skills in releasing the ball. But if he is unable to "see" the ball going through the basket, his success will be limited. Even free-throw shooting skills can be enhanced with visualization and *SportsVision* training.

Table 5.3 outlines a *SportsVision* program for basketball players.

Table 5.3

Basketball SportsVision Training Program

	Week 1	Week 2	Week 3	Week 4	Week 5	Week 6
Focusing	Exercise 3	B	GW	MS	B / GW	B / HM
Tracking	Exercise 4	B	RE	MS	B	B / J
Vergence	Exercise 18	B	GW	HM	MS	B / HM
Coordination	Exercise 25	–	–	–	SL	SL
Coordination	Exercise 39	–	B	MS	MET	B / SL
Visualization	Exercise 46	–	–	–	–	–

Modifications for Basketball

1. Exercise 3, Near–Far Chart (page 40), modified for basketball by placing far chart on backboard or on the ceiling of weight room. Another possibility is partner resistance: Two players stand back to back, and each tries to push the other out of a three-foot-by-three-foot square while performing exercise 3.

2. Exercise 4, Dice Pursuits (page 41), modified for basketball by placing numbers on the basketball rather than using a die. The numbered basketball is shown to the athlete. The coach then throws the ball up in the air and calls out plus or minus. The athlete adds or subtracts the number seen to the running number shown at the start.

3. Exercise 18, Opaque Lifesaver Card (page 53), modified for basketball by taping card to rim of hoop.

4. Exercise 25, Letter Tracking and Ball Bouncing (page 58), modified for basketball by placing letter chart on backboard and focusing on a letter while shooting. The coach can also put letter chart on clipboard and move around floor while moving the clipboard to stimulate eye movements while dribbling and passing.

5. Exercise 39, Flip Sticks (page 69).

6. Exercise 46, Sport-Specific Visualization (page 76), using basketball visualization chart (appendix I.16).

   a. Make free throws without hitting backboard.

   b. Make free throws by banking ball off backboard.

   c. Work on three-point shooting from behind line on court.

7. Group activity: Exercise 50, Arrow Chart (page 80). Perform this at the end of each training session in weeks 1 to 6.

8. *SportsVision* court training:
   a. Color the seams of the basketball with tape of a contrasting color.
   b. Use tach targets during dribbling drills.
   c. Visualize free throws before shooting.
   d. Play five on five using two different colored basketballs (not recommended for youth players).

Boxing

Eye–hand coordination, balance, peripheral awareness, and central awareness are key components of effective boxing. Boxing requires heightened visual skills and the ability to sustain those skills for the entire fight. Fatigue of the visual system can be as costly as muscular fatigue as the match progresses; therefore, the boxer with the better-trained visual system has a distinct advantage in landing punches more accurately. Table 5.4 outlines a *SportsVision* program for boxing.

Modifications for Boxing

1. Exercise 6, Two Strip Saccades (page 42), modified for boxing by putting the saccade strips on coach's boxing gloves. Emphasize foot movement and boxing stance while coach moves gloves in all planes and directions.

2. Exercise 10, Double Bead String Fixations (page 47), modified for boxing by using boxing stance and balance. This exercise can be used as a good prefight warm-up. The boxer fixates from bead to bead as quickly as a punch would come at the boxer.

3. Exercise 18, Opaque Lifesaver Card (page 53), modified for boxing by having coach move card as an opponent's head might move during fight.

4. Exercise 28, Punching O's (page 60), modified for boxing by working on hand quickness and accuracy as in throwing a punch.

Table 5.4
Boxing SportsVision Training Program

	Week 1	Week 2	Week 3	Week 4	Week 5	Week 6
Tracking	Exercise 6	B 🦶	RE	MS 🧍	MS 🏃	PLYO
Tracking	Exercise 10	B ✏️	GW	HM	MS 🏃	MET
Vergence	Exercise 18	B 🖥️	HM	GW	MS 🏃 🚶🚶	PLYO
Coordination	Exercise 28	B �	GW	HM	MS 🏃	B ✏️ B 🎾
Coordination	Exercise 34	HM	GW	B ✏️	B 🖥️ GW	B 🦶 MET
Visualization	Exercise 41	—	—	—	—	—

    a. Another modification is to punch O's not in sequence but rather randomly around the chart.

    b. Be sure to use both right and left hands randomly during exercise, as they are used during a fight.

5. Exercise 34, Bimanual Circles (page 65), modified for boxing by emphasizing balance activities that are as like those in boxing as possible.

6. Exercise 41, Space Matching (page 72), modified for boxing by judging the distance between opponents during a fight to see how well the boxer can judge striking distances.

7. Group activity: Exercise 50, Arrow Charts (page 80), at the end of training session.

8. *SportsVision* training in the ring or gym:

    a. Place letters on heavy bag or speed bag.

    b. Place target points on opponent's headgear for specific places to hit.

    c. Place target points on opponent's body for specific places to hit.

    d. Do as many *SportsVision* exercises as possible while jumping rope.

Cricket

Cricket is one of the most visually demanding sports. Because cricket is played with a very small, high-velocity projectile, binocular vision needs to be optimized. *SportsVision* training can make the cricket player aware of where the ball is in the field and where the ball and the player need to be to make the play. Hitting in cricket is unlike hitting the ball in any other sport, in that the ball is hit after it bounces off the ground. This action demands unique visual skill. Table 5.5 outlines a *SportsVision* training program for cricket.

Table 5.5

Cricket SportsVision Training Program

	Week 1	Week 2	Week 3	Week 4	Week 5	Week 6
Focusing	Exercise 1	B [foot]	B [seesaw]	RE	B [foot] GW	MS [person] [person]
Focusing	Exercise 2	B [seesaw]	RE	B [balls]	HM	B [BAL]
Tracking	Exercise 7	MET	B [seesaw] RE	B [foot] MET	SL	B [trampoline] MET SL
Tracking	Exercise 9	GW	HM	B [balls]	B [BAL]	B [foot] HM
Coordination	Exercise 26	GW	B [seesaw]	B [seesaw] GW	B [seesaw]	B [BAL]
Coordination	Exercise 35	B [trampoline]	B [balls]	SL	B [trampoline] SL	B [balls] SL

Modifications for Cricket

1. Exercise 1, Focusing Pursuits (page 39), modified for cricket by using a ball marked with five different numbers and five different letters. Each number or letter should be approximately half an inch high.

2. Exercise 2, Near–Far Eye Jumps (page 39), modified for cricket by using the same ball as in exercise 1 for the near target.

3. Exercise 7, Ball Batting (page 43), modified for cricket by using a cricket bat.

4. Exercise 9, Bead String (page 46), modified for cricket by making the string equal to the distance from bowler to the wickets (20 meters).

5. Exercise 26, Straw Piercing (page 59).

6. Exercise 35, Beanbags From Behind (page 66).

7. Group activity (can be done by small group or entire team): Exercise 47, VDP Charts (page 78). Perform this at the end of each training session in weeks 1 to 6.

8. *SportsVision* field training:

  a. Color seams on the ball for use in batting practice or during catch.

  b. Put numbers or letters on a ball. See how many characters the athlete can see before hitting or catching the ball.

  c. Play waffle ball under a strobe light, hitting the ball off the bounce and fielding the ball after it has been hit.

  d. Play catch with a tennis ball under a strobe light. Practice throwing balls in the air and catching ground balls.

  e. Bat a tennis ball under a strobe light. Practice hitting the ball off the bounce.

Cycling

A cyclist needs to be able to recognize the hazards of the road ahead. This requires instantaneous visual skills and reaction to environmental conditions. In addition, the cyclist needs to be keenly aware of his position in relationship to his teammates and opponents as the course changes. This requires quick and accurate eye movements, heightened spatial awareness, balance, and visualization of the remainder of the race. Table 5.6 outlines a *SportsVision* training program for cycling.

Modifications for Cycling

1. Exercise 5, Find the Number (page 42), modified for cycling by performing the exercise while

  a. riding a bicycle on a stand;

  b. balancing on the bicycle.

2. Exercise 14, VDP Ball With Thinking (page 50), modified for cycling by doing "abdominal cycling" exercise with lower extremities (lying on your back, pedaling with your feet in the air) during the drill.

3. Exercise 20, Pencil Push-ups (page 54), modified for cycling by performing the exercise while bicycling on a stand, or balancing on the bicycle. This is a good prerace warm-up.

4. Exercise 27, Spaghetti in Straw (page 59), modified for cycling by performing exercise

  a. under variable lighting conditions;

  b. while wearing cycling sunglasses or eyewear.

Table 5.6

Cycling SportsVision Training Program

		Week 1	Week 2	Week 3	Week 4	Week 5	Week 6
Tracking	Exercise 5	B	B BAL	GW	MS / MS	B BAL / SL
Tracking	Exercise 14	RE	MS	GW	HM	RE / HM
Vergence	Exercise 20	B	B	B BAL / GW	HM / MS	HM / MS
Sequencing	Exercise 24	–	–	–	–	–
Coordination	Exercise 27	B	B / HM	HM	B BAL / GW	B / GW HM
Coordination	Exercise 38	B BAL	B / GW	B / MET	OEO	B

5. Exercise 38, Egg Carton Catch (page 68), modified for cycling by performing the exercise while

    a. pedaling a stationary cycle;

    b. pedaling under variable light conditions or wearing cycling eyewear.

6. Group activity: Exercise 49, Ferris Wheel (page 80).

7. *SportsVision* training on the bicycle:

    a. Visualize the course.

    b. Read numbers on license plates while riding on the road.

    c. Perform as many *SportsVision* training exercises as possible while balancing on the bicycle.

Diving

No other sport requires more visualization and balance than diving. The ability to visualize the dive while climbing up the ladder will significantly contribute to the success of the dive. The diver must be able to visualize the target area on the surface of the water and to be aware of and control where she is in space throughout the dive. Diving has unique visualization demands; divers visualize the dive in their mind's eye before actually attempting the dive. A visualized score of 10 has a much higher probability of becoming an actual score of 10. Table 5.7 outlines a *SportsVision* training program for diving.

Table 5.7

Diving SportsVision Training Program

	Week 1	Week 2	Week 3	Week 4	Week 5	Week 6
Tracking	Exercise 9	B [foot]	B [ruler]	HM	B [trampoline]	B [trampoline] GW
Sequencing	Exercise 21	B [trampoline]	B [foot] / B [trampoline]	B [ball]	B [balls] / B [foot]	B [foot] / B [trampoline]
Sequencing	Exercise 23	GW	HM	B [foot] GW	B [trampoline] HM	B [trampoline] GW HM
Coordination	Exercise 29	B [foot]	B [foot] / B [trampoline]	B [screen]	MS [figure]	B [trampoline] HM
Coordination	Exercise 37	B [trampoline]	B [screen]	B [board] GW	PLYO	GW PLYO
Visualization	Exercise 46	B [trampoline]	B [balls]	B [ball]	J SL	B [trampoline] / J HM

Modifications for Diving

1. Exercise 9, Bead String (page 46), modified for diving by attaching string to end of board and having athlete stand on board during exercise.

2. Exercise 21, Auditory Span With Vision (page 56).

3. Exercise 23, Picture Memories (page 57).

4. Exercise 29, Penny Drop (page 60).

5. Exercise 37, Broomstick Balancing (page 67).

6. Exercise 46, Sport-Specific Visualization (page 76), modified for diving by closing eyes and drawing movement pattern of each dive.

7. Group activity: Exercise 48, Simon Says (page 79).

8. *SportsVision* training in the pool:

   a. Do exercise 21, Auditory Span With Vision, with coach calling out number sequence while athlete dives. Diver must repeat sequence on returning to pool deck.

Downhill Skiing

Effective recreational or competitive skiers must master the visual ability to see the next three turns ahead. Although this may sound like a fairly simple process, it can be quite challenging. Once the skier makes the first turn, she has to be able to see three more turns ahead. If the skier plans only for the next turn, the visual motor system has no way to prepare in time to actually complete that next turn. Balance also plays a key role in skiing, and on crowded slopes, even the recreational skier can benefit from peripheral awareness activities to decrease the chance of collision with another skier. Table 5.8 outlines a *SportsVision* training program for skiing.

Table 5.8

Downhill Skiing SportsVision Training Program

	Week 1	Week 2	Week 3	Week 4	Week 5	Week 6
Tracking	Exercise 12	B 🦶	B 🛹	HM	B 📺 / GW	B 🛏 / J
Tracking	Exercise 16	MS 🧍	B 🛹	B 📺	GW	PLYO / MS 🦵
Coordination	Exercise 31	OEO	B 🛹	B 🦶 / GW	HM / SL	B 🛏 / HM SL
Coordination	Exercise 39	B 🛹	B 🦶	B 🦶 / HM	MS 🧍 / B 🛏	PLYO / MS 🦵
Visualization	Exercise 41	–	–	–	–	–
Visualization	Exercise 46	B 🛏	B 🎾	B 🔵	B 🛹	B 🛏 / HM

Modifications for Downhill Skiing

1. Exercise 12, Four-Square Chart Fixations (page 48), modified for skiing by putting charts on giant slalom gates.

    a. Perform balance loading activities while wearing ski boots.

2. Exercise 16, Slow Pursuits (page 51), modified for skiing by using tip of ski pole as a target.

    a. Do the exercise while riding chair lift; use targets such as oncoming chairs, oncoming poles, other skiers coming down the mountain.

3. Exercise 31, Continuous Motion (page 62), modified for skiing by drawing numbered gates on chalkboard.

    a. Perform balance loading activities while wearing ski boots.

4. Exercise 39, Flip Sticks (page 69), modified for skiing by using actual ski poles for the catching sticks.

5. Exercise 41, Space Matching (page 72), modified for skiing by estimating distances between two slalom poles.

6. Exercise 46, Sport-Specific Visualization (page 76), modified for skiing as follows:

    a. Skier closes eyes, and coach holds red or blue gate in front of skier.

   b. Skier opens eyes and must move right for a red gate or left for a blue gate. This exercise can be done in the training facility or even on the slopes prior to the race.

7. Group activity: Exercise 48, Simon Says (page 79), performed on balance board. After the board touches the ground five times, the skier is out.

8. *SportsVision* training on the slopes:

   a. Do eye movement activities while on the chair lift.

   b. Visualize the course before the race.

Figure Skating

Figure skating demands optimal balance, visualization, and eye movement accuracy. Developing balance with eye movement, head movement, and gaze work activities is critical to success in this sport. The inability to focus while spinning can be a limiting factor for some skaters. The exercises and loading variations for figure skating specifically address the visual demands of this sport. Table 5.9 outlines a *SportsVision* training program for figure skating.

Modifications for Figure Skating

1. Exercise 2, Near–Far Eye Jumps (page 39).

2. Exercise 11, Flashlight Chase (page 48), modified for figure skating by tracing the path of the skating routine with the flashlights.

3. Exercise 22, Hand Sequencing (page 56).

4. Exercise 37, Broomstick Balancing (page 67), modified for figure skating by performing the exercise while skating at the rink.

Table 5.9

Figure Skating SportsVision Training Program

	Week 1	Week 2	Week 3	Week 4	Week 5	Week 6
Focusing	Exercise 2	B	B	B / GW	B / HM	B / HM MET
Tracking	Exercise 11	MS	MS	B	MS / SL	B / B
Sequencing	Exercise 22	—	—	—	—	—
Coordination	Exercise 37	B	B / HM	B / GW	GW / SL	B / OEO
Visualization	Exercise 40	MET	MET	HM / MET	MET / SL	HM / MET SL
Visualization	Exercise 43	B	B	B	B / GW	B / GW

5. Exercise 40, Delayed Memory (page 71).

6. Exercise 43, Parquetry Patterns (page 74).

7. Group activity: Exercise 47, VDP Charts (page 78).

8. *SportsVision* training on the ice:

    a. Do exercise 3, Near–Far Chart (page 40), with coach skating backward holding the near chart. The skater then focuses on a peripheral object (e.g., advertisement on boards) and alternates reading near chart held by coach with far object while skating.

    b. Do exercise 6, Two-Strip Saccades (page 42), while skating. Coach holds the chart and skates backward as skater performs the routine and calls out letters as soon as she sees them. *Note:* Do not cut two-chart page down the middle. Leave as one page!

    c. Do exercise 50, Arrow Chart (page 80). Coach skates backward holding arrow chart while skater identifies with hands up, down, right and left.

Football

The tremendous visual demands of football vary by the specific needs and activities of the different positions. Vision, balance, tracking, eye movements, peripheral awareness, eye–hand coordination, and near–far focusing are all required in football. Ball handlers can significantly improve their performance with *SportsVision*, but our work with the U.S. Air Force Academy has demonstrated that even interior linemen can benefit from *SportsVision* training. Table 5.10 outlines a *SportsVision* training program for football.

Table 5.10

Football SportsVision Training Program

	Week 1	Week 2	Week 3	Week 4	Week 5	Week 6
Focusing	Exercise 3	B [foot]	J	RE	MS [icon] MS [icon]	B [balls] HM MET
Tracking	Exercise 4	RE	B [board]	B [ball]	J	B [foot] B [ball]
Vergence	Exercise 18	HM	GW	B [icon]	MS [icon]	B [icon] RE HM
Coordination	Exercise 36	B [board]	B [trampoline]	MS [icon] HM	SL	HM SL
Coordination	Exercise 39	OEO	B [foot]	MS [icon]	HM	B [board] SL
Visualization	Exercise 42	B [foot]	OEO	HM	MS [icon] MET	B [ball] GW

Modifications for Football

1. Exercise 3, Near–Far Chart (page 40), modified for football by putting letters on football for use as near chart.

2. Exercise 4, Dice Pursuits (page 41), modified for football by having a partner push or pull player's body or otherwise distracting player.

3. Exercise 18, Opaque Lifesaver Card (page 53), modified for football by performing exercise in weight room between sets.

4. Exercise 36, Juggling (page 66), modified for football by using

    a. small footballs;

    b. regular size footballs;

    c. footballs of different sizes.

5. Exercise 39, Flip Sticks (page 69), modified for football by

    a. wearing helmets and pads while performing exercise;

    b. performing exercise while walking through a pattern (e.g., pulling guard, short receiver route).

6. Exercise 42, Quick Exposure (page 73), modified for football by putting plays on each card.

7. Group activity: Exercise 47, VDP Charts (page 78).

8. *SportsVision* field training:

    a. Place letters or numbers on the ball.

    b. Place letter charts on blocking sleds.

    c. Use tach targets during blocking drills.

    d. Coach bounces football on ground, and athlete has to catch it before it bounces a given number of times (two to five bounces).

Golf

The visual demands of golf are so great that an entire textbook has been written on the subject (Farnsworth 1997). Golf is unique in that while many sports involve hitting a moving object, golf requires the athlete to hit a small, stationary object. Although this may sound significantly easier, anyone who has ever tried to hit that little white ball out of six inches of rough with a downhill lie knows that it is not as easy as it sounds. Technology has dramatically improved the distance and accuracy of most golfers' shots. But one of the major advances in professional golf is golf-specific strength and conditioning programs. The most successful professional golfers today include sports vision training in their overall conditioning program. Although *SportsVision* training may not help you drive the ball over 300 yards, it can definitely help lower your score and improve your enjoyment of the game. Table 5.11 outlines a *SportsVision* training program for golf.

Modifications for Golf

1. Exercise 9, Bead String (page 46), modified for golf by

    a. tying string to flag on practice green.

    b. performing exercise while in golf stance.

    c. String should be approximately 40 feet long.

Table 5.11

Golf SportsVision Training Program

	Week 1	Week 2	Week 3	Week 4	Week 5	Week 6
Tracking	Exercise 9	B ⬚	B ⬚	GW	HM	B ⬚ GW
Coordination	Exercise 27	OEO	GW	HM	B ⬚	MS ⬚
Coordination	Exercise 34	B ⬚	B ⬚⬚	B ⬚	GW	B ⬚ HM
Coordination	Exercise 39	OEO	B ⬚	MS ⬚⬚	SL	HM SL
Visualization	Exercise 41	–	–	–	–	–
Visualization	Exercise 46	–	–	–	– SL	– SL

2. Exercise 27, Spaghetti in Straw (page 59).

3. Exercise 34, Bimanual Circles (page 65).

4. Exercise 39, Flip Sticks (page 69), modified for golf by using two old clubs for the catching sticks.

5. Exercise 41, Space Matching (page 72), modified for golf by estimating the distance of putts on the putting green.

6. Exercise 46, Sport-Specific Visualization (page 76), modified for golf by

   a. playing against an opponent;

   b. playing by golf rules regarding hazards, out-of-bounds, and so on;

   c. having to "play" ball out of trap laterally, not forward.

7. *SportsVision* training on the course:

   a. Juggle golf balls while waiting.

   b. Tap ball with club face, keeping ball in the air.

   c. "Putt" ball with driver closest to tee marker while waiting to tee off.

Gymnastics

Gymnastics combines vision, eye–hand coordination, visualization, and balance in a dynamic setting. It is necessary for a gymnast to be aware of his overall body scheme, unlike most other athletes. The interaction between eye movements, body positioning, peripheral awareness, and eye movement skills are critical in all gymnastics events. Gymnastics is a unique sport in which visual acuity (20/20 vision) is not a key component to success; however, because gymnastics is a highly visual sport, performance can be improved through the *SportsVision* program outlined in table 5.12.

Table 5.12

Gymnastics SportsVision Training Program

	Week 1	Week 2	Week 3	Week 4	Week 5	Week 6
Tracking	Exercise 12	B [foot]	B [stick]	J	B [foot] OEO	B [stick] GW
Vergence	Exercise 17	B [stick]	MS [person] MS [person]	OEO	B [BAL]	B [balls]
Sequencing	Exercise 22	–	–	–	–	–
Coordination	Exercise 36	B [foot] OEO	B [stick] SL	B [trampoline] HM	B [BAL] HM SL	B [tv] OEO SL
Coordination	Exercise 37	RE	GW	RE HM	MS [person] SL	RE MS [person]
Visualization	Exercise 43	–	–	–	–	–

Modifications for Gymnastics

1. Exercise 12, Four-Square Chart Fixations (page 48), modified for gymnastics by placing charts around gym.

2. Exercise 17, Near–Far Rocking (page 52), modified for gymnastics by placing far chart on vaulting horse.

3. Exercise 22, Hand Sequencing (page 56).

4. Exercise 36, Juggling (page 66).

5. Exercise 37, Broomstick Balancing (page 67).

6. Exercise 43, Parquetry Patterns (page 74).

7. Group activity: Exercise 48, Simon Says (page 79).

8. *SportsVision* training in the gym:

   a. Coach holds a tach target while walking around the apparatus, and the athlete must correctly identify the target.

   b. Place various letter and/or number charts around the gym, and the athlete looks for and then calls out the appropriate letter and/or number at different points in the routine.

   c. Place charts on landing areas to help the athlete first visually find and then focus or concentrate on sticking the landing in that specific area.

Hockey

Talk about the ultimate visual sport! The velocity and density of the hockey puck far exceed those of any other small projectile used in other sports. The hockey goalkeeper needs to be able to see and track a small rubber puck that can travel up to 120 miles per hour in a slap shot. The other players need to judge the speed and direction of the puck, attempt to control the puck using a four-inch-wide blade, change directions, and then either pass to an open teammate or shoot to the opening in the net to score. All this is accomplished on an incredibly slippery surface while five other players try to knock you off your feet to take you out of the play. This sport combines vision and balance, focusing, eye–hand coordination, tracking, and eye movements. Table 5.13 outlines a *SportsVision* training program for hockey.

Table 5.13

Hockey SportsVision Training Program

	Week 1	Week 2	Week 3	Week 4	Week 5	Week 6
Focusing	Exercise 2	B 🦶	B 🪵	J	B 🦶 / OEO	B 🪵 / GW
Tracking	Exercise 8	B (BAL)	GW	HM	GW / HM	B 🪵 / MET
Vergence	Exercise 18	B 🪵	B (BAL)	GW	HM	MS 🧍 / MS 🧍↔🧍
Coordination	Exercise 35	OEO	MS 🚶	HM	HM / MS 🚶	PLYO / SL
Coordination	Exercise 37	B 🦶	B 🪵	RE	GW / SL	B ⚫⚫ / SL
Visualization	Exercise 42	—	—	—	—	—

Modifications for Hockey

1. Exercise 2, Near–Far Eye Jumps (page 39), modified for hockey by using a puck for near focus and the goal for far focus.

2. Exercise 8, Ball Tap (page 45), modified for hockey by putting a puck on a string and tapping the puck with hockey stick. Modify further by performing the exercise with puck at different heights.

3. Exercise 18, Opaque Lifesaver Card (page 53).

4. Exercise 35, Beanbags From Behind (page 66), modified for hockey by using a puck and wearing helmet and glove.

5. Exercise 37, Broomstick Balancing (page 67), modified for hockey by balancing the hockey stick.

6. Exercise 42, Quick Exposure (page 73).

7. Group activity: Exercise 47, VDP Charts (page 78).

8. *SportsVision* training on the ice:
   a. Coach uses tach targets during practice.
   b. Put four-square charts (Appendix I.9) on the four corners of the goal.
   c. Put numbers on the puck for quick eye movements for the goalkeeper.
   d. Put near chart on puck (Appendix I.3, slightly larger letters) and far chart on goal for individual stick-handling drills.
   e. One player wears a number or different colored vest. All players must be aware of where the marked player is. The coach gives the command "Freeze" and asks where the marked player is: right, left, behind, or in front, or closest to which line.

Lacrosse

Lacrosse combines the speed of hockey, the field dimensions of soccer, and the visual demands of football. The visual demands of the sport are enormous. The ability to track the rock-hard projectile requires quick eye movements, near–far focusing, and balancing skills. The lacrosse player must be able to catch and throw the ball with sticks of various sizes that can just as likely be used as "weapons." In addition, protective headgear is required for men's lacrosse. The face mask dramatically affects the athletes' ability to see peripherally. Consequently, athletes benefit from *SportsVision* peripheral vision exercises performed while wearing their headgear. Table 5.14 outlines a *SportsVision* training program for lacrosse.

Table 5.14

Lacrosse SportsVision Training Program

	Week 1	Week 2	Week 3	Week 4	Week 5	Week 6
Focusing	Exercise 2	B	B	OEO	B / OEO	B / GW
Tracking	Exercise 8	B	GW	HM	OEO / HM	B / MET
Vergence	Exercise 18	B	B BAL	GW	HM	MS / MS / MS
Vergence	Exercise 19	B	B BAL / MS	GW	HM	MS / MS
Coordination	Exercise 35	B	B / OEO	GW / MS	GW / SL	B / SL
Coordination	Exercise 39	B	B	MS	GW / SL	B / SL

Modifications for Lacrosse

1. Exercise 2, Near–Far Eye Jumps (page 39), modified for lacrosse by using a stick and the goal for the near and far points.

2. Exercise 8, Ball Tap (page 45), modified for lacrosse by using a lacrosse stick for tapping a lacrosse ball duct-taped to the string.

3. Exercise 18, Opaque Lifesaver Card (page 53).

4. Exercise 19, Hot Dog in the Sky (page 54).

5. Exercise 35, Beanbags From Behind (page 66), modified for lacrosse by using a lacrosse stick to catch a lacrosse ball.

   a. Use two balls.

   b. Player closes eyes and waits for the coach's command "now" to open eyes.

6. Exercise 39, Flip Sticks (page 69), modified for lacrosse by using two lacrosse sticks as catching sticks.

7. Group activity: Exercise 47, VDP Charts (page 78).

8. *SportsVision* field training:

   a. Coach uses tach targets.

   b. Coach places targets in different parts of the goal.

      i. Train without goalkeeper.

      ii. Train with goalkeeper.

   c. Selected players wear different colored vests.

      i. Other players must pass to a marked player before the shot.

      ii. The marked player acts as "man-up" player.

Racket Sports

Racket sports such as badminton, racquetball, squash, and tennis have similar visual demands. Therefore, we provide one training program for all racket sports. The major differences in the four racket sports are the size of the ball, the size of the court, and the lighting contrasts between indoor and outdoor racket sports. Coaches and athletes are encouraged to use the racket and ball for their sport where appropriate in the training program described in table 5.15.

Modifications for Racket Sports

1. Exercise 3, Near–Far Chart (page 40), modified for racket sports by putting near chart on racket and far chart on wall or net.

2. Exercise 5, Find the Number (page 42), modified for racket sports by placing numbers at farthest distance possible on court.

3. Exercise 7, Ball Batting (page 43), modified for racket sports by placing sheet with numbers on face of racket and hitting ball with number called out by coach.

4. Exercise 17, Near–Far Rocking (page 52).

5. Exercise 30, Decode Chart (page 61), modified for racket sports by assigning these actions to the symbols:

   a. Circle: Bounce down.

   b. Square: Bounce up.

Table 5.15

Racket Sport SportsVision Training Program

	Week 1	Week 2	Week 3	Week 4	Week 5	Week 6
Focusing	Exercise 3	GW	HM	MS	MS	B HM
Tracking	Exercise 5	B	OEO	GW	OEO HM	B OEO SL
Tracking	Exercise 7	B	OEO	GW	HM	B MET SL
Vergence	Exercise 17	MS	HM MS	GW MS	B	B HM
Coordination	Exercise 30	–	–	–	–	– GW
Coordination	Exercise 36	B	OEO	MS	B HM	B GW SL

    c. Triangle: Bounce down and then up.

    d. Rectangle: Bounce against the wall.

  6. Exercise 36, Juggling (page 66), modified for racket sports by bouncing sport-specific ball on racket.

    a. Use two balls.

    b. Use two balls and two rackets.

    c. Use three balls with one or two rackets.

  7. Group activity: Exercise 50, Arrow Chart (page 80).

  8. *SportsVision* training on the court:

    a. Color seams of ball.

    b. Put numbers on ball.

    c. Serve to specific target points on court.

    d. Coach uses tach targets to teach how to "hit it where they aren't."

Rugby

Rugby presents several interesting challenges for *SportsVision* training. Although the visual skills needed for rugby are similar to American football, every player on a rugby side is a potential ball handler and therefore needs to work on peripheral awareness, near–far focusing, and tracking skills. Rugby players also suffer a significant number of eye injuries due to the lack of head protection and consequently many rugby players require some form of eye protection after an eye injury. Table 5.16 outlines a *SportsVision* training program for rugby.

Table 5.16

Rugby SportsVision Training Program

	Week 1	Week 2	Week 3	Week 4	Week 5	Week 6
Focusing	Exercise 3	B	J	RE	MS / MS	B / HM MET
Tracking	Exercise 4	RE	B	B (BAL)	J	B / B
Vergence	Exercise 18	HM	GW	B	MS	B / RE HM
Coordination	Exercise 36	B	B	MS	SL	HM / SL
Coordination	Exercise 39	OEO	B	MS	HM	B / SL
Visualization	Exercise 42	B	OEO	HM	MS / MET	B / GW

Modifications for Rugby

1. Exercise 3, Near–Far Chart (page 40), modified for rugby by putting letters on ball and putting far chart 10 to 20 feet away on wall or goalpost.

2. Exercise 4, Dice Pursuits (page 41), modified for rugby by having a partner push or pull player's body or otherwise distracting player.

3. Exercise 18, Lifesaver Card (page 53), modified for rugby by performing exercise in weight room between sets.

4. Exercise 36, Juggling (page 66), modified for rugby by using

   a. small rugby balls;

   b. regular size rugby balls;

   c. rugby balls of different sizes.

5. Exercise 39, Flip Sticks (page 69).

6. Exercise 42, Quick Exposure (page 73), modified for rugby by putting plays on each card.

7. Group activity: Exercise 47, VDP Charts (page 78).
8. *SportsVision* training on the field:
   a. Place letters or numbers on the ball.
   b. Coach uses tach targets during practice.
   c. Coach bounces rugby ball on ground, and athlete has to catch it before it bounces a given number of times (two to five bounces).

Soccer

Soccer provides a unique challenge to the visual system in that good eye–foot and eye–head coordination is needed by all players except the goalkeeper. Soccer also involves visualization skills similar to skiing: The better soccer players know what they are going to do with the ball three or four moves ahead of time. Soccer requires the athlete to see the field and the opponent but also the open space for passing lanes or for shots into the goal. The vast majority of shots, even in the professional ranks, are right at the goalkeeper because the goalkeeper's colorful jersey is usually the last thing the player sees before taking the shot. *SportsVision* training helps players to see not where the goalkeeper is, but rather where the goalkeeper is *not* and helps them make more goals and have more fun. Table 5.17 outlines a *SportsVision* training program for soccer.

Modifications for Soccer

1. Exercise 2, Near–Far Eye Jumps (page 39), modified for soccer as follows:
   a. Put numbers on ball. Athlete calls out number before kicking ball.
   b. Put numbers on goal net in various locations.

Table 5.17

Soccer SportsVision Training Program

	Week 1	Week 2	Week 3	Week 4	Week 5	Week 6
Focusing	Exercise 2	B [foot]	OEO	RE	MS [runner] / MS [lunge]	B [balls] / HM
Tracking	Exercise 15	B [board]	B [trampoline]	OEO	HM	B [foot] / OEO
Vergence	Exercise 18	HM	GW	MS [runner] / RE	MS [runner] / MS [lunge]	B [monitor] / HM
Vergence	Exercise 19	HM	GW	MS [runner]	MS [runner] / MS [lunge]	B [monitor] / HM
Coordination	Exercise 37	B [foot]	B [foot] / HM	B [board] / GW	B [balls] / SL	B [foot] / HM SL
Visualization	Exercise 46	—	—	—	—	—

    i. Coach calls out number, and athlete kicks ball at that number on the net.

    ii. Athlete calls out number while kicking ball.

2. Exercise 15, Saccade Column Movements (page 51), modified for soccer by performing exercise while

    a. dribbling ball;

    b. performing "quick feet" foundations;

    c. juggling soccer ball with feet.

3. Exercises 18 and 19, Opaque Lifesaver Card (page 53) and Hot Dog in the Sky (page 54), modified for soccer by performing exercise while

    a. dribbling ball;

    b. performing "quick feet" foundations;

    c. juggling soccer ball with feet.

4. Exercise 37, Broomstick Balancing (page 67), modified for soccer by

    a. attempting to balance broomstick on foot. Be sure to practice this balance exercise using each foot.

    b. attempting to balance soccer ball on foot. Be sure to practice this balance exercise using each foot.

    c. attempting to balance broomstick on hand and soccer ball on foot.

5. Exercise 46, Sport-Specific Visualization (page 76), using soccer goal visualization chart (appendix I.20).

    a. Practice penalty kick with eyes closed.

    b. Practice free kick over wall with eyes closed.

    c. Practice corner kick with eyes closed.

6. Group activity: Exercise 47, VDP Charts (page 78).

7. *SportsVision* field training:

    a. Place numbers or letters on ball, and call out number before heading ball to coach or teammate.

    b. Place numbers or letters on ball for practice curving ball when kicking.

    c. Place numbers on field marking cones for better field awareness.

    d. Selected players wear different-colored vests. Other players must play ball to one of those players before shot in goal.

    e. Coach uses tach targets during dribbling drills, juggling drills, and controlled scrimmage situations to get players to look up more during game.

Volleyball

Success in volleyball is based on the simple premise of hitting the ball where the opponent isn't. This is more difficult than it sounds. *SportsVision* improves peripheral awareness to see where teammates are, near–far focusing to see where openings on the opponent's side of the net are, and eye–hand coordination for hitting the ball at the right place and time. Table 5.18 outlines a *SportsVision* training program for volleyball.

Table 5.18

Volleyball SportsVision Training Program

	Week 1	Week 2	Week 3	Week 4	Week 5	Week 6
Tracking	Exercise 10	MS	MET	GW	HM	B HM
Tracking	Exercise 14	OEO	RE	GW	HM	RE HM
Vergence	Exercise 18	B	J	HM	MS MS	B HM
Vergence	Exercise 19	B	J	HM	MS MS	B HM
Coordination	Exercise 32	B	B	B	OEO	MS SL
Coordination	Exercise 36	B	B	MS	SL MS	B SL

Modifications for Volleyball

1. Exercise 10, Double Bead String Fixations (page 47), modified for volleyball by tying the string to the top of the volleyball net.

2. Exercise 14, VDP Ball With Thinking (page 50), modified for volleyball by putting numbers on the volleyball. Coach spins volleyball, and players try to follow a given number while answering questions.

3. Exercises 18 and 19, Opaque Lifesaver Card (page 53) and Hot Dog in the Sky (page 54).

4. Exercise 32, Catcho (page 63), modified for volleyball by using a volleyball rather than a beanbag.

5. Exercise 36, Juggling (page 66), with volleyballs.

   a. Once players can juggle volleyballs, they juggle different balls (e.g., tennis balls, softballs).

6. Group activity: Exercise 50, Arrow Chart (page 80).

7. *SportsVision* training on the court:

   a. Place numbers or letters on volleyball.

   b. Place specific targets on floor to hit during spiking drills.

   c. Coach uses tach targets during practice to help players see where opponents will be during games.

   d. Players on receiving side keep eyes closed until the coach calls out, "Open eyes." This teaches players to track ball more rapidly.

   e. Play volleyball with strobe light; use a Nerf ball or soft volleyball to start.

APPENDIXES

Four-in-One Balance Beam Construction Guide

Materials:

(1) 4″ × 4″ × 8′ board for main balance beam

(1) 2″ × 2″ × 6′ board for attached balance beam

(1) 1″ × 2″ × 6′ board for attached balance beam

(1) 1″ diameter × 6′ dowel for attached balance beam

(2) 2″ × 8″ × 2′ boards for base

(4) 2″ × 8″ × 10″ boards for beam support on base

(31) 2 3/4″ wood screws

Sandpaper

Construction:

a. Cut the 8″ wide boards to length.

b. Attach the four 2″ × 8″ × 10″ boards with four wood screws each to the 2″ × 8″ × 2′ board base so there is a 3 1/2″ space for a balance beam in the middle 2″ × 8″ × 2′ base of the four 2″ × 8″ × 10″ boards.

c. Mark 1′ from each end on each of the four surfaces of the 4″ × 4″ × 8′ board.

d. Attach the 2″ × 2″ × 6′ board parallel to the main balance beam (the 4″ × 4″ × 8′ board) along the middle of one surface, between the 1′ marks, with five wood screws.

e. Similarly attach the 1″ × 2″ × 6′ board to middle of another surface with five wood screws.

f. Similarly attach the 1″ diameter × 6′ dowel to middle of a third surface with five wood screws.

g. Sand all surfaces.

 From *SportsVision* by Thomas A. Wilson and Jeff Falkel, 2004, Champaign, IL: Human Kinetics.

SportsVision Screening Evaluation Form

Name: _____ Age: _____ Before: _____ After: ___

Sport/position: _____ Date: _____

1. Focusing

	Trial 1	Trial 2	Trial 3	Average
Near–far chart Exercise 3 (Score: Letters per minute)	_____	_____	_____	_____

2. Tracking

	Trial 1	Trial 2	Trial 3	Average
Two-strip saccades Exercise 6 (Score: Letters per minute)	_____	_____	_____	_____

3. Vergence

	Trial 1	Trial 2	Trial 3	Average
Pencil push-ups Exercise 20 (Score: Inches)	_____	_____	_____	_____

4. Sequencing

	Trial 1	Trial 2	Trial 3	Average
Hand sequencing Exercise 22 (Score: Largest sequence completed correctly)	_____	_____	_____	_____

5. Eye–hand coordination

	Trial 1	Trial 2	Trial 3	Average
Egg carton catch Exercise 38 (Score: Seconds)	_____	_____	_____	_____

6. Visualization

	Trial 1	Trial 2	Trial 3	Average
Ace to Seven Exercise 45 (modified) (Score: Seconds)	_____	_____	_____	_____

From *SportsVision* by Thomas A. Wilson and Jeff Falkel, 2004, Champaign, IL: Human Kinetics.

Hand Sequencing
Pre- and Posttraining Form

P S F

F P S F

S F P S P

F S F P F S

P P S F S F P

S F P F P S F P

F F P S P S F P F

S P F P S P F P S P

P = Palm   S; = Side of Hand;   F = Fist

   From *SportsVision* by Thomas A. Wilson and Jeff Falkel, 2004, Champaign, IL: Human Kinetics.

Teeter Board Construction Guide

Materials

(1) 15″ × 18″ × 3/4″ plywood for balance platform

(1) 15″ × 2″ × 3/4″ hardwood for teeter beam

(5) 2 1/2″ wood screws

Sandpaper

Nonskid surface material

Construction

1. Cut plywood to size.

2. Cut hardwood teeter beam to size.

3. Attach hardwood teeter beam to middle of plywood balance platform with wood screws.

4. Sand plywood base and teeter beam.

5. Attach nonskid surface material to balance platform.

Parquetry Pattern Template

Parquetry patterns can be made of very thick poster board or a product of similar weight. They can also be purchased at specialty toy stores or academic supply stores.

1. Cut out four identical 3″ × 3″ squares.
2. Cut two of the squares in half diagonally to make four isosceles triangles.
3. Cut out two identical 4″ × 1 1/2″ rectangles.
4. Various shapes can be made, as long as they are made in pairs of equal size and shape. A different color for each shape is recommended. The exact dimensions are not critical, as long as both partners have identical matching pieces.
5. Here are examples of five different shapes that can be cut out and replicated.

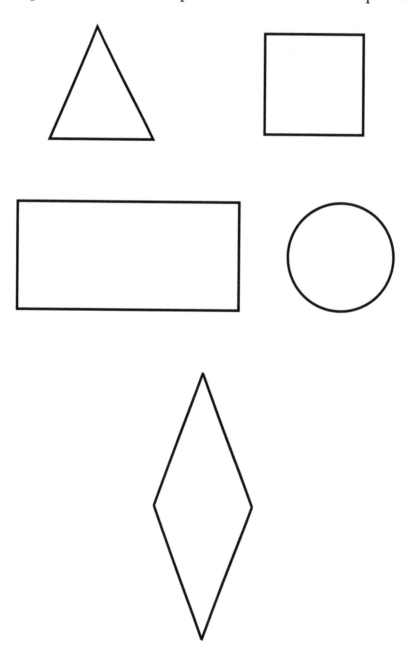

From *SportsVision* by Thomas A. Wilson and Jeff Falkel, 2004, Champaign, IL: Human Kinetics.

Equipment Manufacturers

EFI
7755 Arjons Dr.
San Diego, CA 92126
800-541-4900
EFI is the distributor of the MFT multifunctional balance apparatus.

Ball Dynamics International
14215 Mead St.
Longmont, CO 80504
800-752-2255
Ball Dynamics is the distributor of the Gymnic® ball, used for loading and balance training.

M-F Athletic Company (Perform Better)
P.O. Box 8090
Cranston, RI 02920
800-556-7464
M-F is a distributor of various balance and functional training apparatuses that can be used for *SportsVision* training.

OEP Foundation
1921 E. Carnegie Ave., Ste. 3-L
Santa Ana, CA 92705
949-250-8070
OEP is the distributor of the lifesaver cards.

Power Systems
P.O. Box 31709
Knoxville, TN 37930
800-321-6975
Power Systems is a distributor of various balance and functional training apparatuses that can be used for *SportsVision* training.

SportsVision Exercise Log Forms

SportsVision Exercise Log

Name: _____ Sport: _____ Week: _____

	Day 1	Day 2	Day 3	Day 4	Day 5
Exercise 1	_____	_____	_____	_____	_____
Exercise 2	_____	_____	_____	_____	_____
Exercise 3	_____	_____	_____	_____	_____
Exercise 4	_____	_____	_____	_____	_____
Exercise 5	_____	_____	_____	_____	_____
Exercise 6	_____	_____	_____	_____	_____

SportsVision Exercise Log

Name: _____ Sport: _____ Week: _____

	Day 1	Day 2	Day 3	Day 4	Day 5
Exercise 1	_____	_____	_____	_____	_____
Exercise 2	_____	_____	_____	_____	_____
Exercise 3	_____	_____	_____	_____	_____
Exercise 4	_____	_____	_____	_____	_____
Exercise 5	_____	_____	_____	_____	_____
Exercise 6	_____	_____	_____	_____	_____

From *SportsVision* by Thomas A. Wilson and Jeff Falkel, 2004, Champaign, IL: Human Kinetics.

Tach Targets

This appendix will provide coaches with a series of letters, numbers, shapes, and objects that they can use in the field to assist their athletes in developing and enhancing sports vision. A tachistoscope is an instrument used to determine the shortest exposure capable of making a conscious impression on the retina. We are using this principle in developing and enhancing sports vision on the field with this book.

To use the book for sports vision training on the field is very simple. There are several sections, each with four variations: letters, numbers, shapes, arrows, and number sequences. During warm-up drills, skill sessions, and even game situations, the coach can hold up a tach target; the athlete should look around for the object while concentrating on the skill or movement involved in the sport. This very basic activity will dramatically improve the athletes' ability to see more on the field or court, and enhance their ability to incorporate more visual awareness into their playing.

There are several other variations that can be used with the tach targets. For example, after holding up several targets, ask the athlete to recite the previous one, rather than the one that is being shown. In the number sequence, have the athlete only call off the middle number, or the end numbers, or the numbers in reverse order (right to left). In addition to the figures and shapes included here, you can use solid sheets of colored paper as targets; ask the athlete to call out the color. The variations are endless, and limited only by the practice environment and the coach's imagination.

Good luck and have fun with these tach targets!

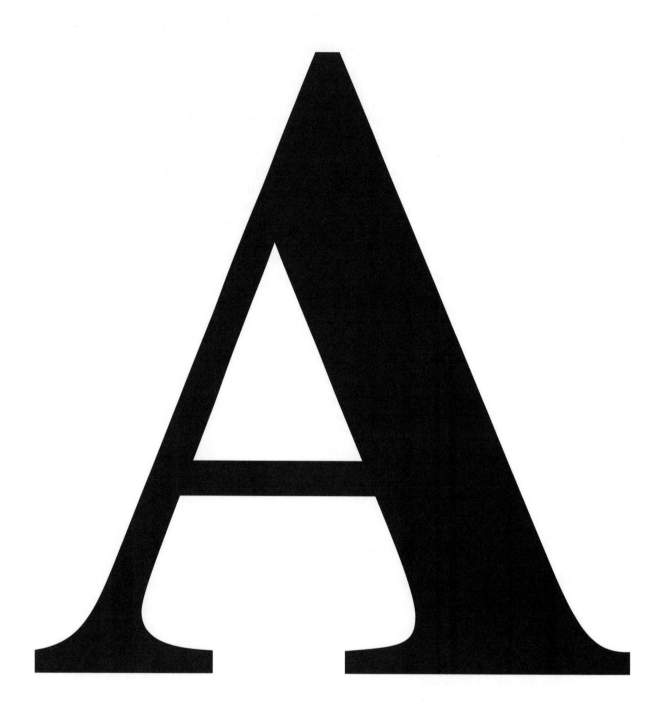

H.2   From *SportsVision* by Thomas A. Wilson and Jeff Falkel, 2004, Champaign, IL: Human Kinetics.

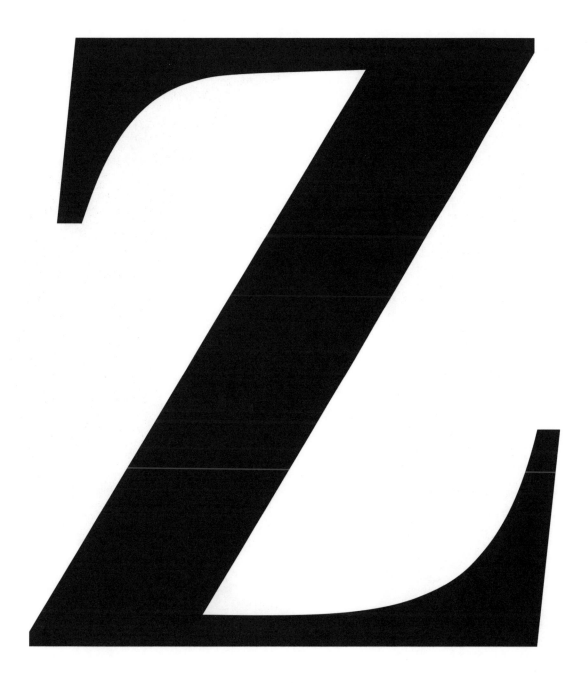

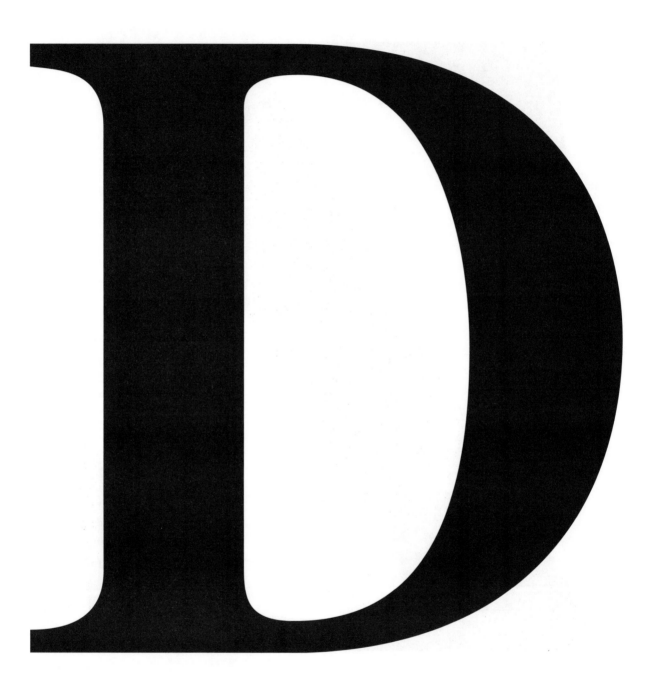

From *SportsVision* by Thomas A. Wilson and Jeff Falkel, 2004, Champaign, IL: Human Kinetics.

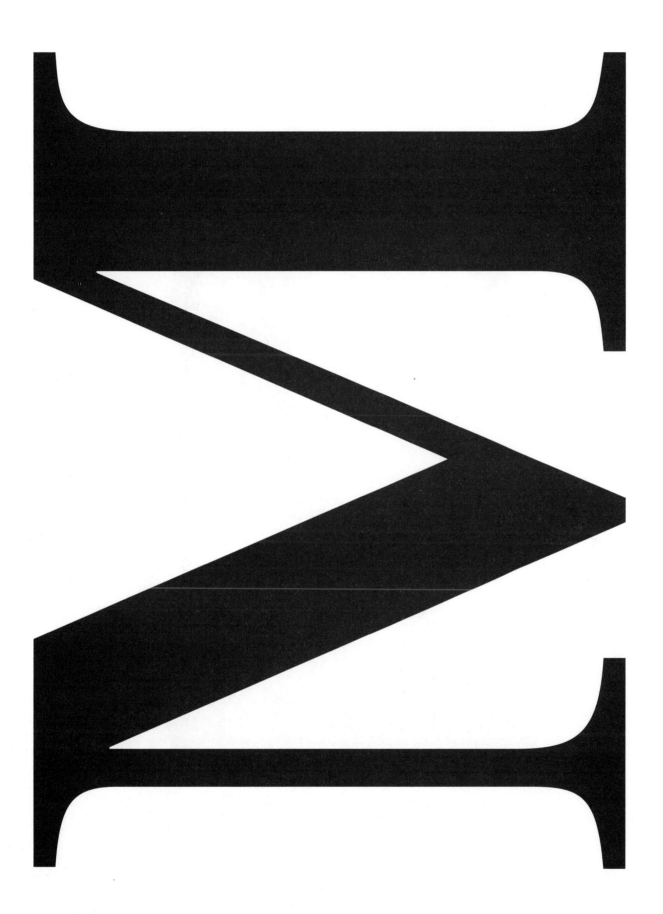

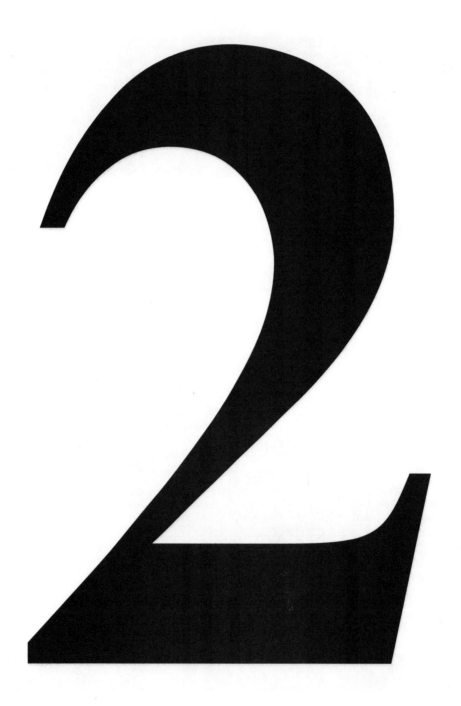

From *SportsVision* by Thomas A. Wilson and Jeff Falkel, 2004, Champaign, IL: Human Kinetics.

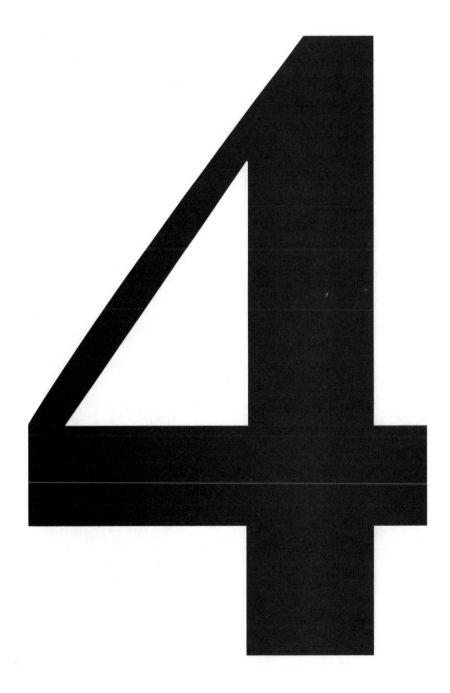

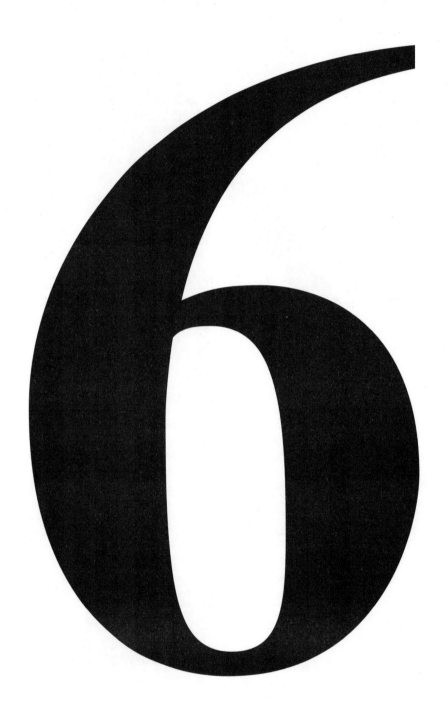

From *SportsVision* by Thomas A. Wilson and Jeff Falkel, 2004, Champaign, IL: Human Kinetics.

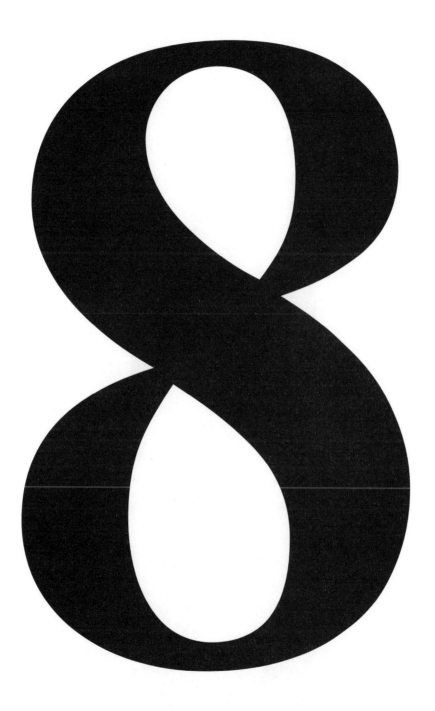

H.9

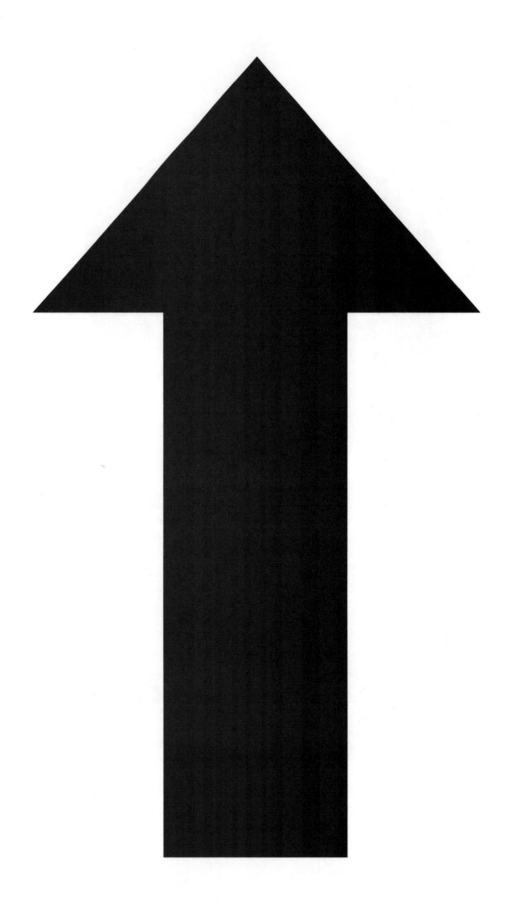

From *SportsVision* by Thomas A. Wilson and Jeff Falkel, 2004, Champaign, IL: Human Kinetics.

H.11

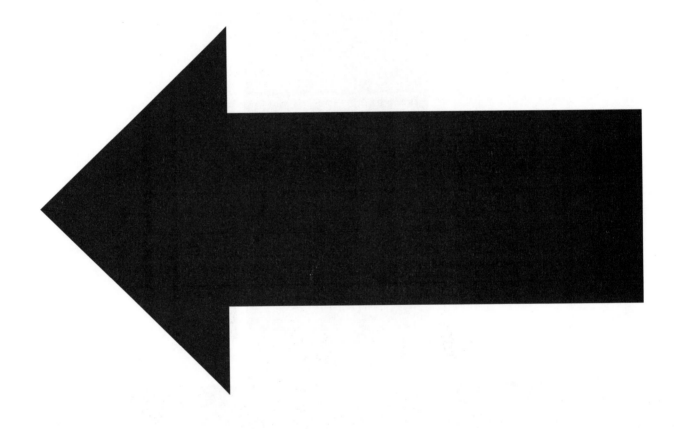

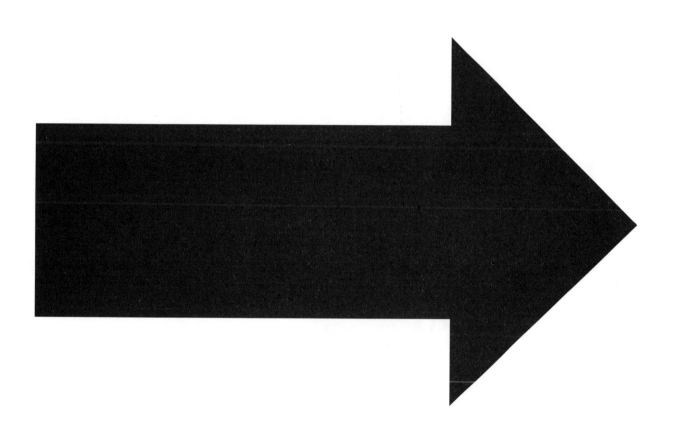

H.13

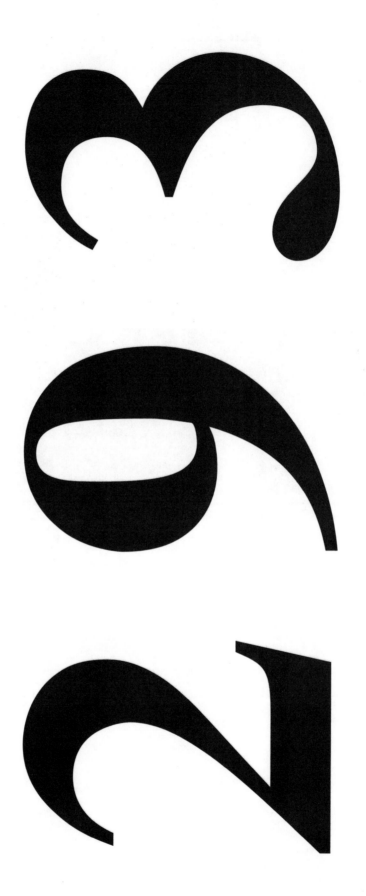

From *SportsVision* by Thomas A. Wilson and Jeff Falkel, 2004, Champaign, IL: Human Kinetics.

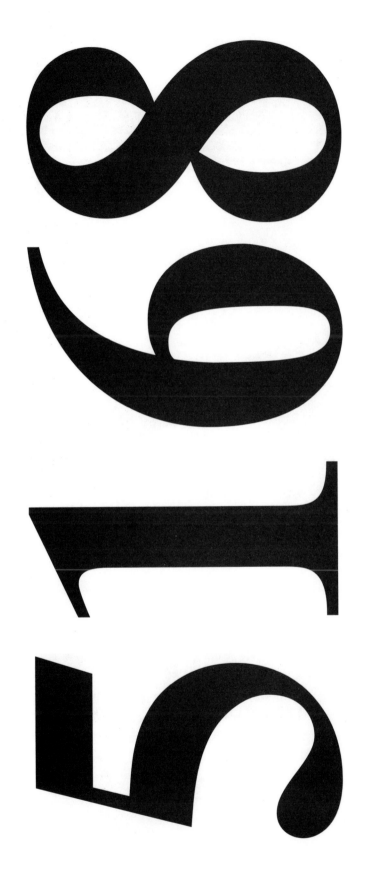

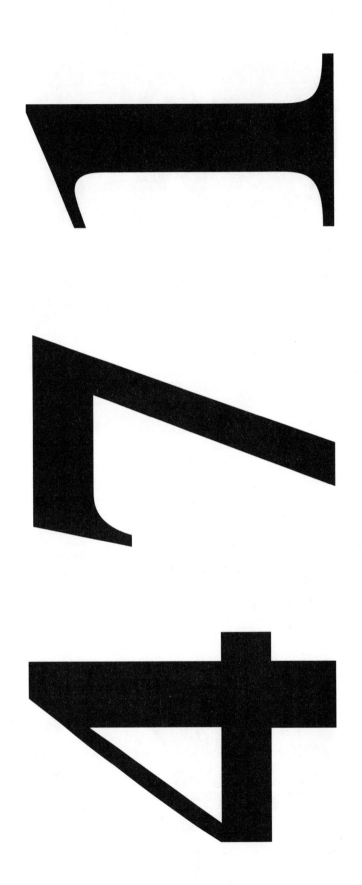

From *SportsVision* by Thomas A. Wilson and Jeff Falkel, 2004, Champaign, IL: Human Kinetics.

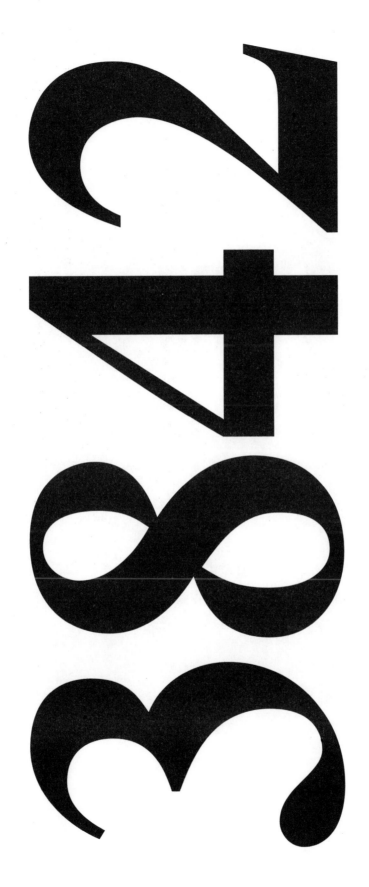

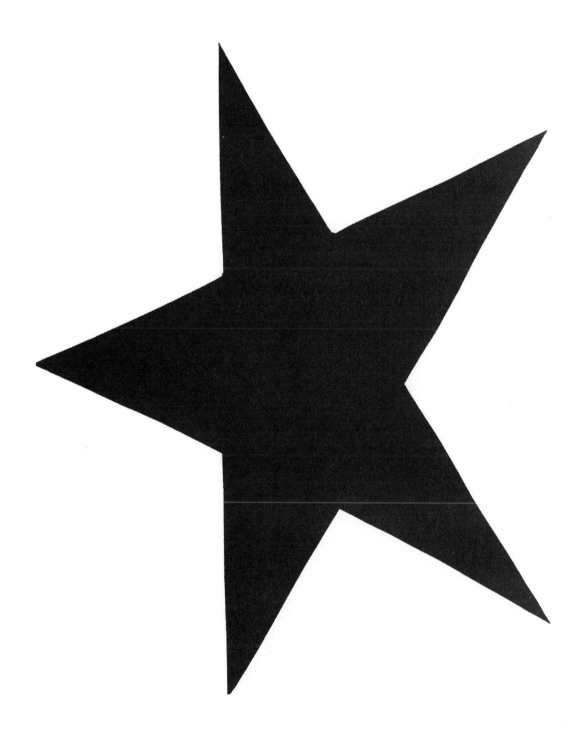

From *SportsVision* by Thomas A. Wilson and Jeff Falkel, 2004, Champaign, IL: Human Kinetics.

H.21

Reproducible Figures and Charts

| 20/40 | Y | N | S | I |
| 20/40 | Z | T | X | A |

20/20	U	H	E	T	A	I
20/20	C	Y	W	Z	F	N
20/20	L	V	D	P	T	A

20/10	Y	H	G	I	P	N
20/10	T	A	W	J	E	F
20/10	C	M	F	T	N	G
20/10	H	R	X	U	O	C

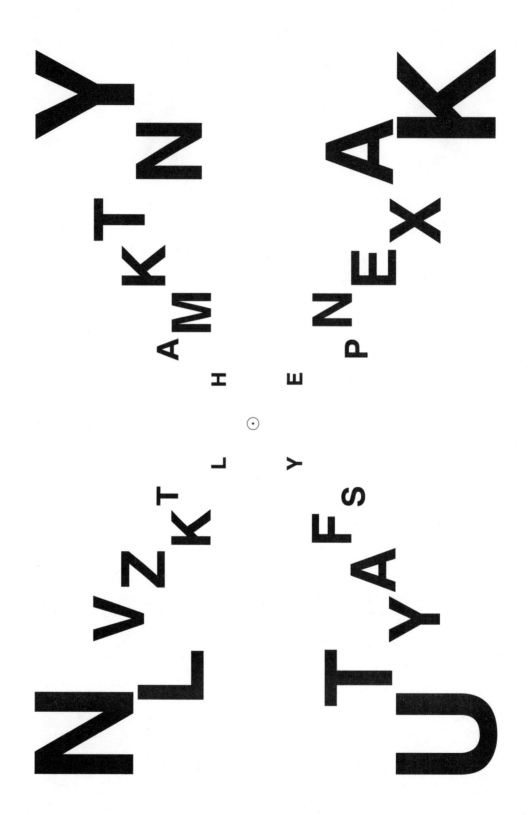

From *SportsVision* by Thomas A. Wilson and Jeff Falkel, 2004, Champaign, IL: Human Kinetics.

W C U I F V C D X S

G F R E S X Z O N T

V S X D Z B H E M Z

Y T E S X J B T O P

E S A Z W Y T D K V

I O N P B Y C D T Z

A V B E Z Y G K J X

K N H B V C X Z R F

T R I H F W A S G K

T R E W Q A Z X C V

A Z R E U O B P L J

S F H K M B C Z Q D

Q W E R T Y U I O P

K L J G H F G D S A

A Z X S W E D C R J

H G F D S A Z X C B

P O U Y T R E W Q M

N J U B H Y T G V D

A S D F G H J K L Q

Z X C V B N M L K J

F D E Q A T Y O P W

G U H B T O V R A J

T Y B C D S A Z O K

E H A J K B V L M D

W Q Z E C N L J H P

M H J U T F C Z A P

T F V H A N C D E W

A D E G J M O X Z T

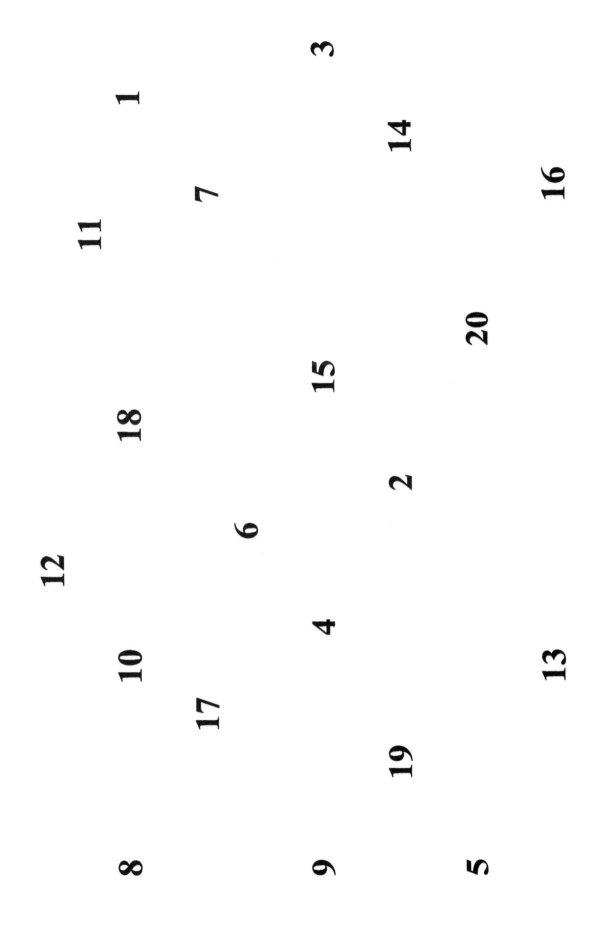

From *SportsVision* by Thomas A. Wilson and Jeff Falkel, 2004, Champaign, IL: Human Kinetics.

I.5

Z		N
O		H
R		F
T		A
C		M
Y		B
U		P
S		I
X		K
N		Q
W		Z
I		J
N		V

 From *SportsVision* by Thomas A. Wilson and Jeff Falkel, 2004, Champaign, IL: Human Kinetics.

B	E
F	K
T	J
Z	Q
P	G
M	I
L	H
X	R
A	U
D	S
N	Y
V	F
X	O
C	T
J	F
A	W
B	Y

C
F
D
R
L
M
O
X
Y
N
Z
K
J
P
A
D
L
Q
Z
T
J
C
G
Y
R

B
X
E
J
P
I
Q
G
K
S
H
U
W
M
Z
C
K
I
P
A
F
M
B
H
Z

A	B	G	8
O	4	6	→
9	↓	F	T
K	5	T	V

T	R	7	↑
5	P	4	M
H	B	←	Z
J	A	7	S

7	P	G	0
↑	E	4	N
2	R	X	A
U	8	←	X

Y	S	3	U
X	I	L	2
B	T	↓	A
6	N	9	→

W   9

E   P

5   A

C   B

T   7

Y   S

2   G

D   Z

R   4

8   J

M   3

From *SportsVision* by Thomas A. Wilson and Jeff Falkel, 2004, Champaign, IL: Human Kinetics.

ARGH J PMYBDVXT

RTGVAMCBCZAKO

ZHFSZUVMCPBAC

TREWQCUNBFRDU

AUDNHRCXPNZXY

TABXEFTMKGZXN

VCRUNPAXZPSAT

ASDFGHJKLPOUY

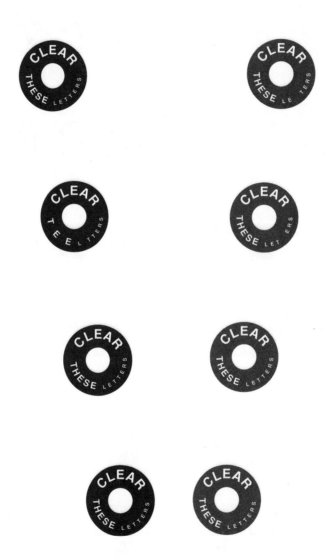

From *SportsVision* by Thomas A. Wilson and Jeff Falkel, 2004, Champaign, IL: Human Kinetics.

o o o o o o o o o o o o o o

o o o o o o o o o o o o o o

o o o o o o o o o o o o o o

o o o o o o o o o o o o o o

o o o o o o o o o o o o o o

o o o o o o o o o o o o o o

o o o o o o o o o o o o o o

o o o o o o o o o o o o o o

o o o o o o o o o o o o o o

o o o o o o o o o o o o o o

o o o o o o o o o o o o o o

o o o o o o o o o o o o o o

o o o o o o o o o o o o o o

o o o o o o o o o o o o o o

o o o o o o o o o o o o o o

o o o o o o o o o o o o o o

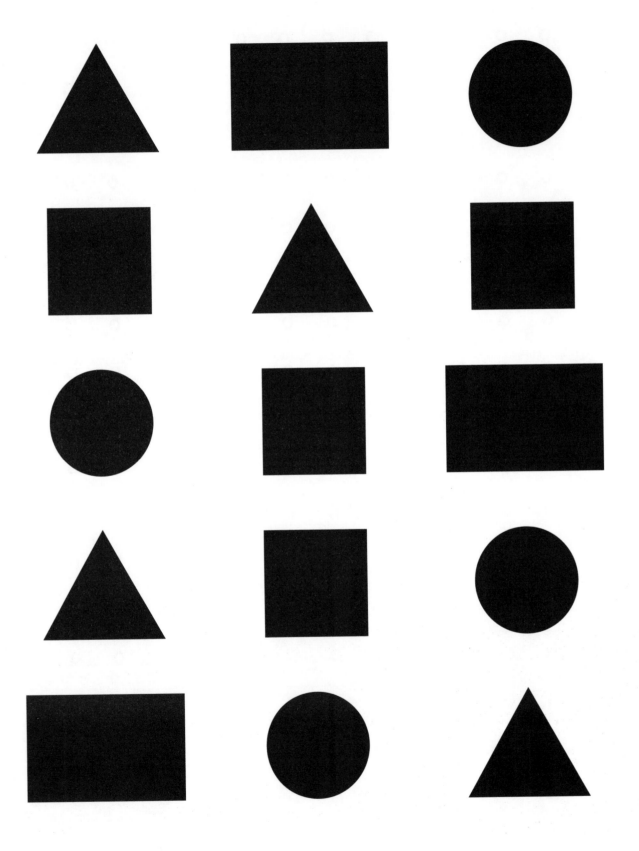

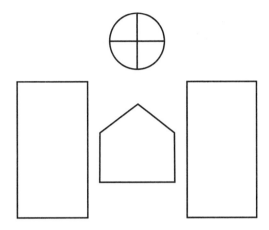

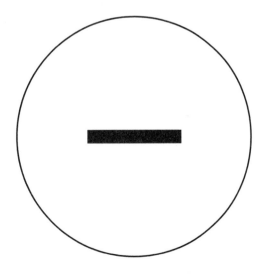

From *SportsVision* by Thomas A. Wilson and Jeff Falkel, 2004, Champaign, IL: Human Kinetics.

I.15

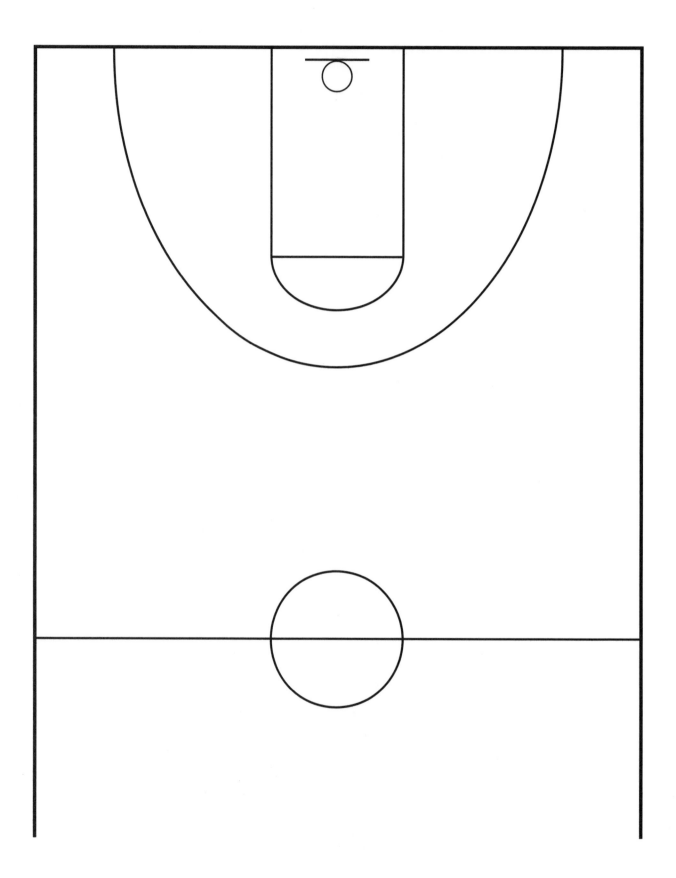

From *SportsVision* by Thomas A. Wilson and Jeff Falkel, 2004, Champaign, IL: Human Kinetics.

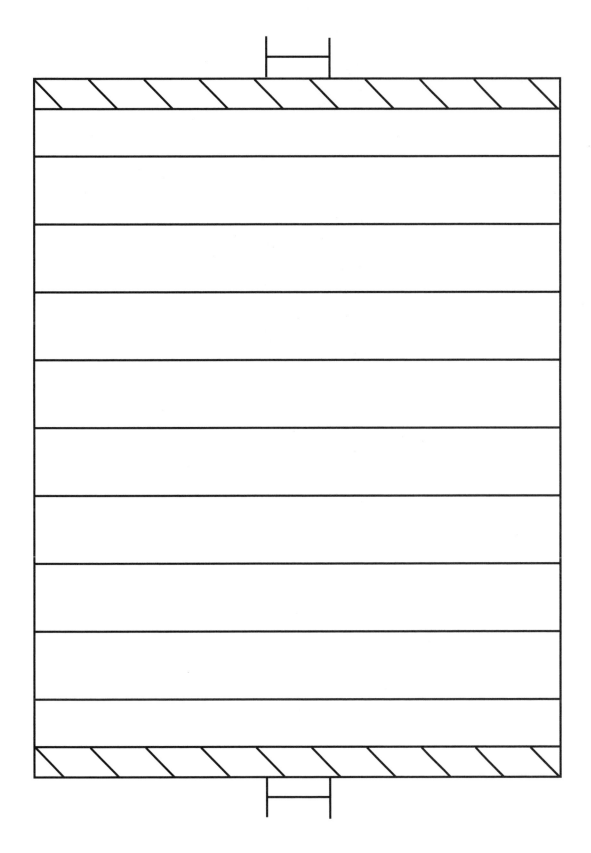

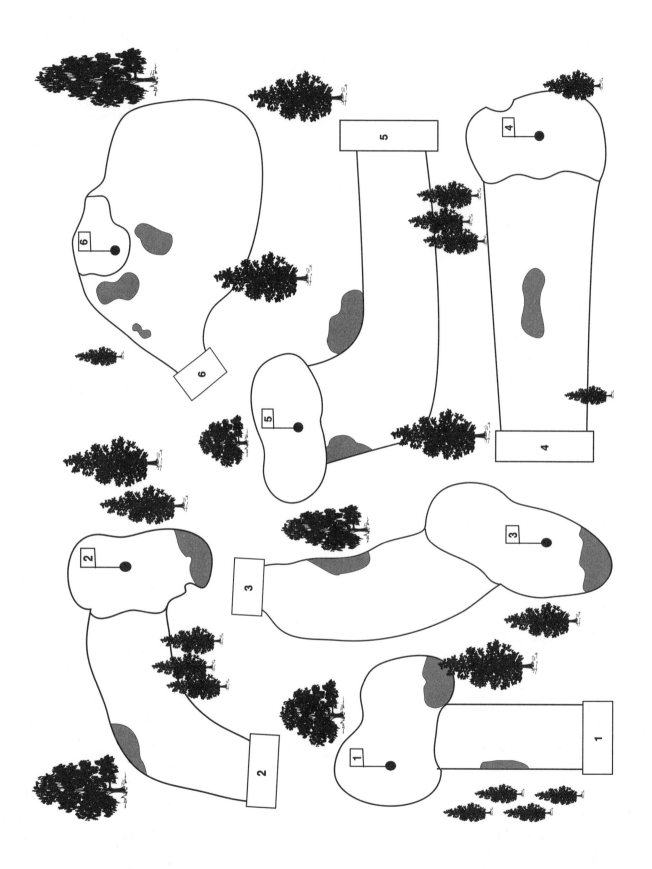

From *SportsVision* by Thomas A. Wilson and Jeff Falkel, 2004, Champaign, IL: Human Kinetics.

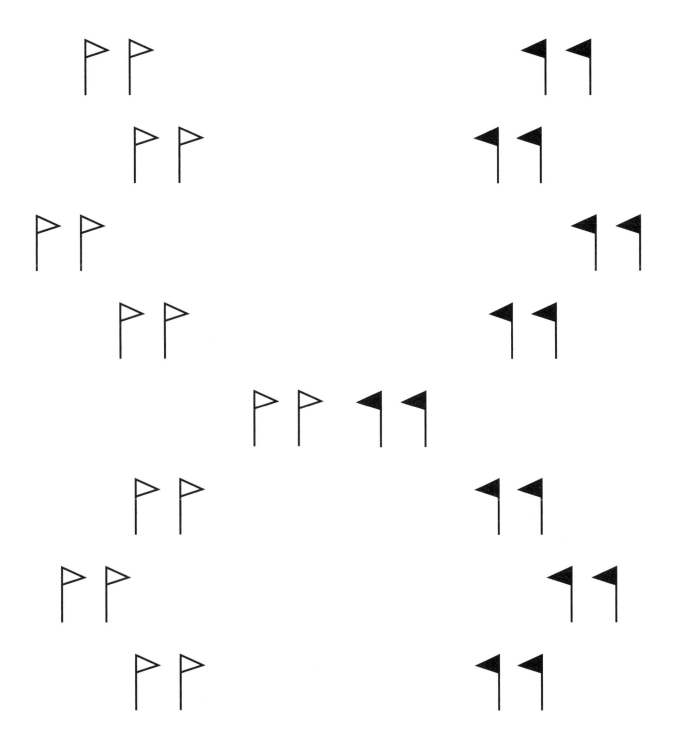

From *SportsVision* by Thomas A. Wilson and Jeff Falkel, 2004, Champaign, IL: Human Kinetics.

I.19

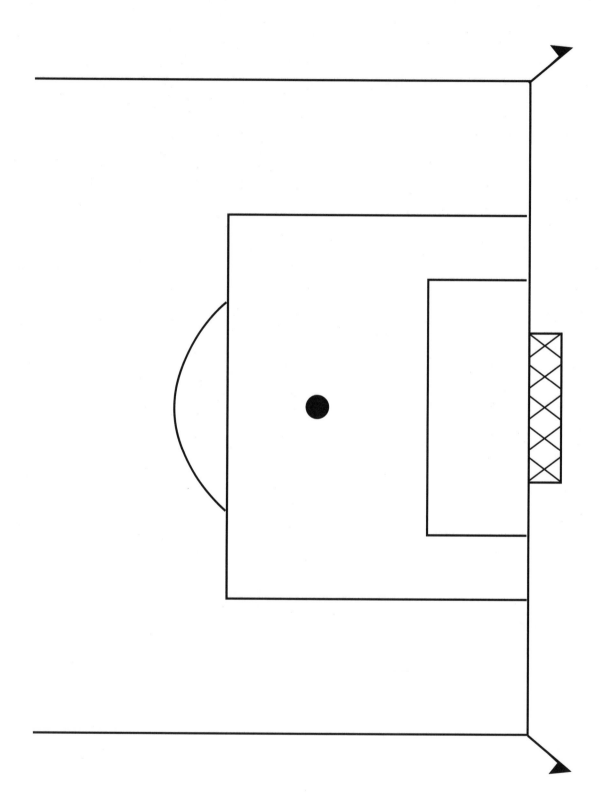

From *SportsVision* by Thomas A. Wilson and Jeff Falkel, 2004, Champaign, IL: Human Kinetics.

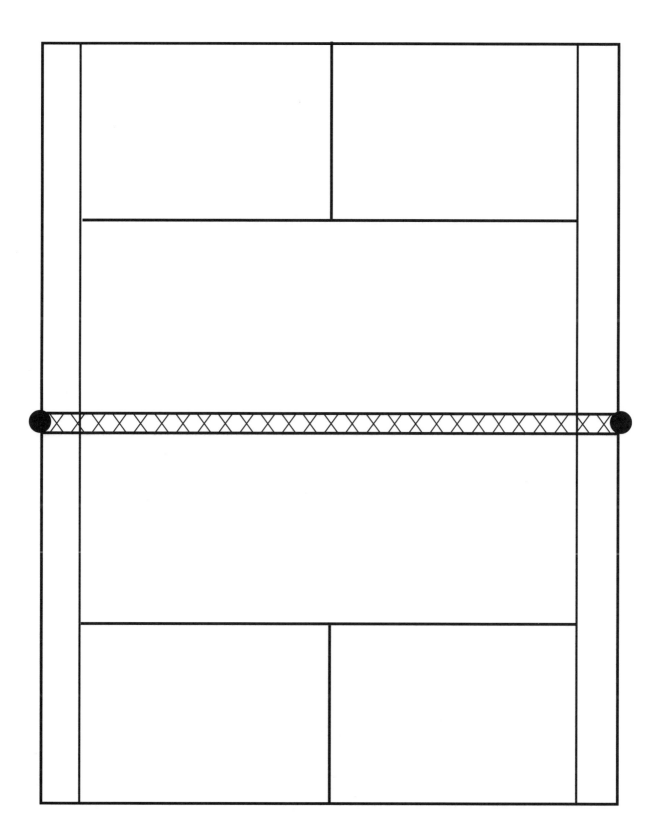

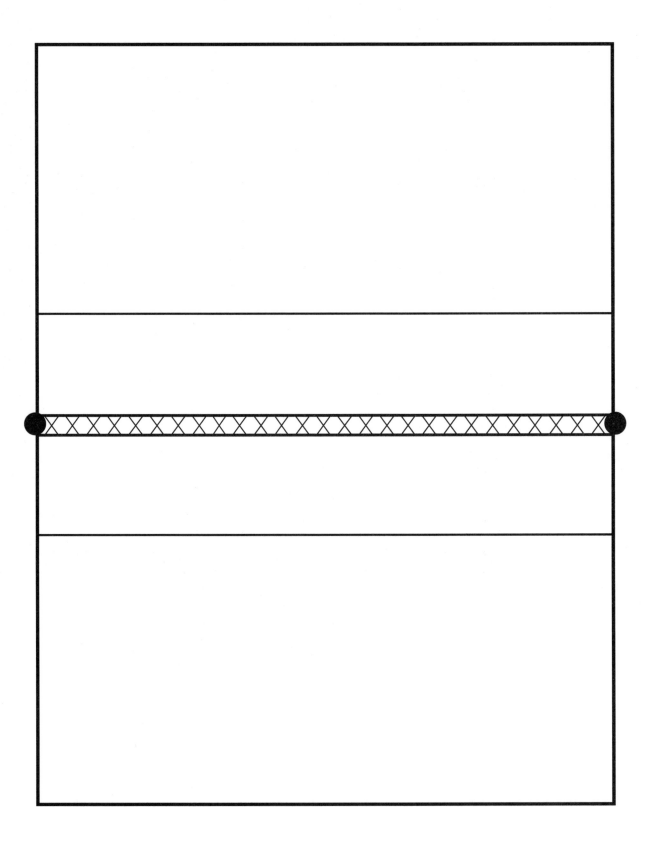

From *SportsVision* by Thomas A. Wilson and Jeff Falkel, 2004, Champaign, IL: Human Kinetics.

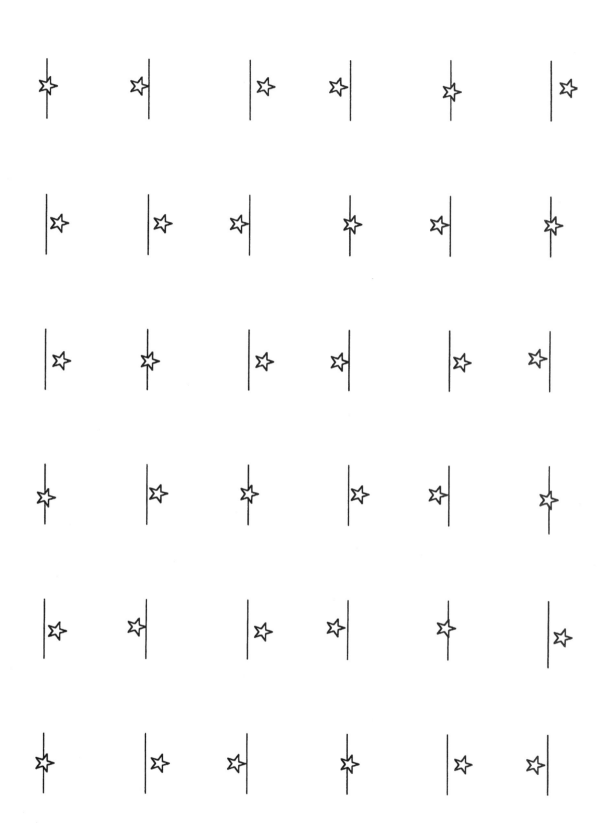

From *SportsVision* by Thomas A. Wilson and Jeff Falkel, 2004, Champaign, IL: Human Kinetics.

I.23

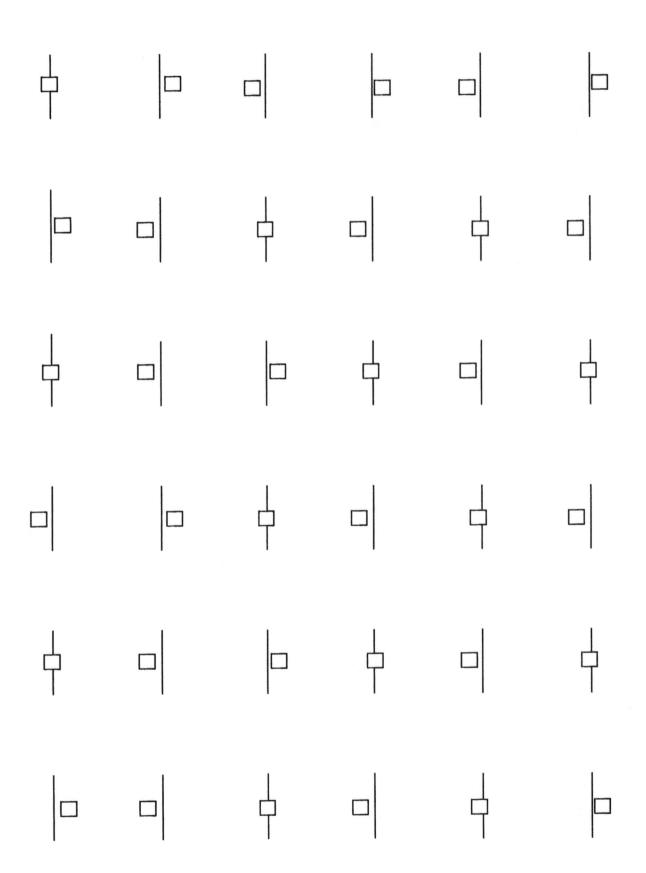

From *SportsVision* by Thomas A. Wilson and Jeff Falkel, 2004, Champaign, IL: Human Kinetics.

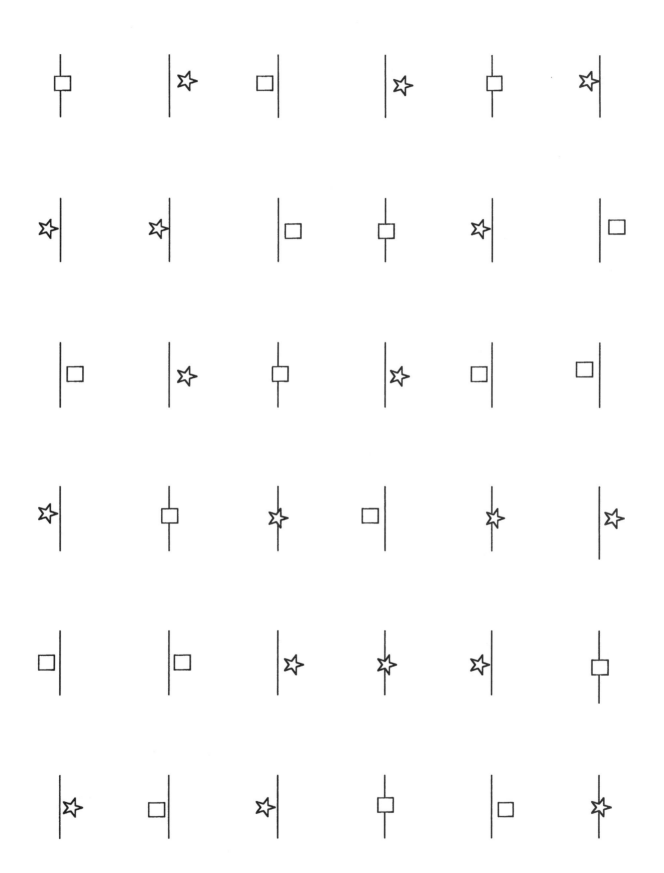

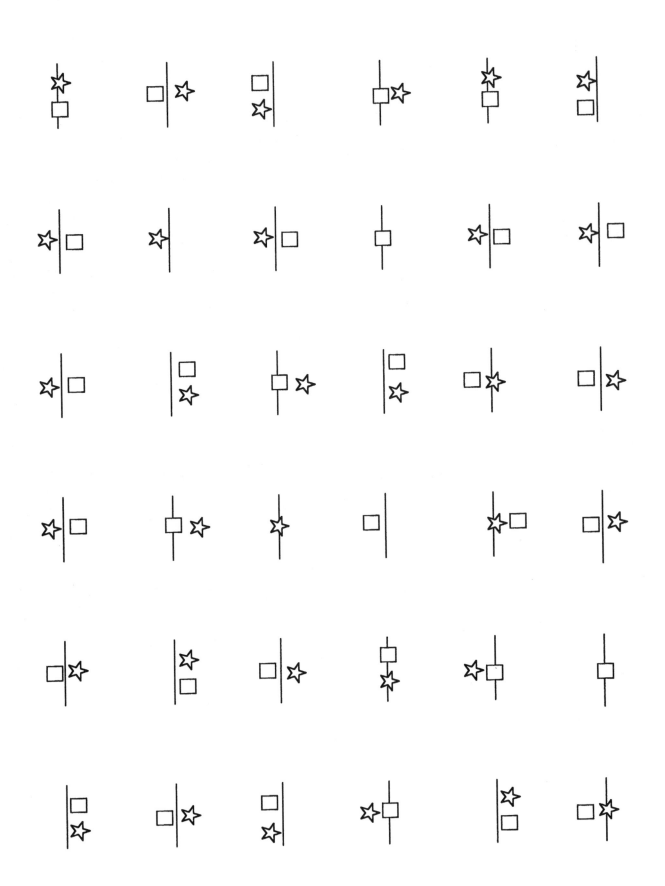

From *SportsVision* by Thomas A. Wilson and Jeff Falkel, 2004, Champaign, IL: Human Kinetics.

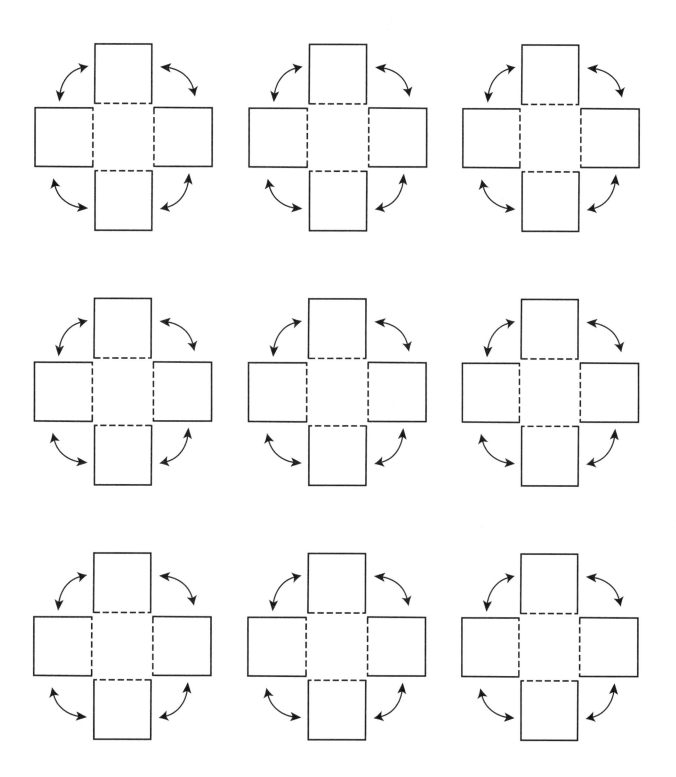

From *SportsVision* by Thomas A. Wilson and Jeff Falkel, 2004, Champaign, IL: Human Kinetics.

I.27

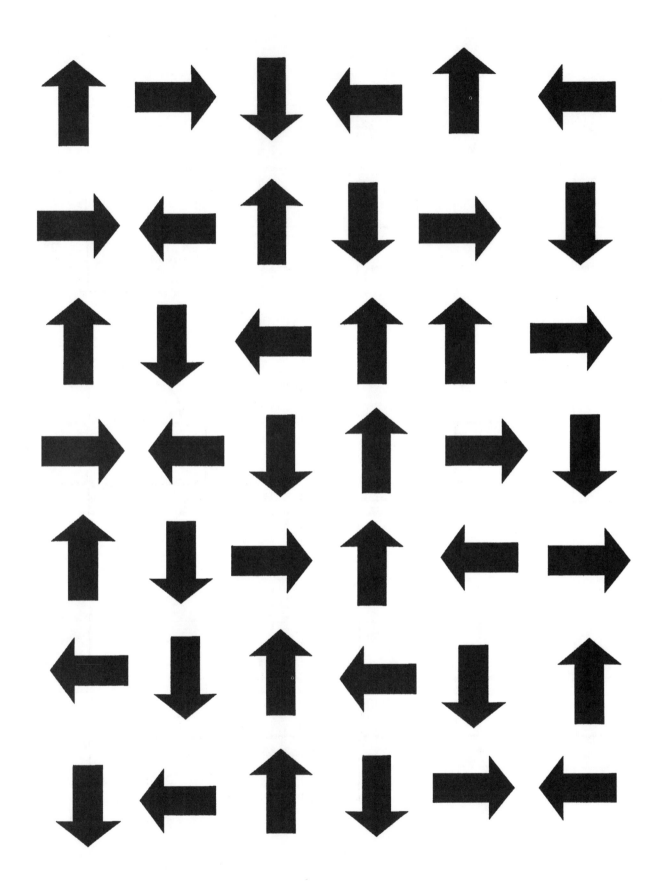

From *SportsVision* by Thomas A. Wilson and Jeff Falkel, 2004, Champaign, IL: Human Kinetics.

BIBLIOGRAPHY

Adolphe, R.M., Vickers, J.M., and Laplante, G. 1997. The effects of training visual attention on gaze behavior and accuracy: A pilot project. *International Journal of Sports Vision* 4 (1): 29–34.

Beckerman, S., and Fornes, A.M. 1997. Effects of changes in lighting level on performance with the AcuVision 1000. *Journal of the American Optometric Association* 68 (4): 243–249.

Brisco, E. 1994. Six principles for making sports vision work. *Review of Optometry* 131 (11): 29–32.

Carlsson, J., ed. 1984. *American optometric sports vision guidebook.* St. Louis: American Optometric Association.

Castellano, C.F. 1996. Visual considerations for the golf enthusiast. *Sports Vision* 12 (3): 10–14.

Chu, D.A. 1998. *Jumping into plyometrics.* Champaign, IL: Human Kinetics.

Classe, J., ed. 1993. *Sports vision.* Norwalk, CT: Appleton and Lange.

Cockerill, I.A., and Macgillivary, W.W. 1981. *Vision and sport.* Cheltenham, England: S. Thornes.

Copeland, V. 1996. Maximizing visual performance for cyclists. *Sports Vision* 12 (2): 23–24.

Davis, R.A. 1994. Make your practice a winner with sports vision. *Optometric Management* 29 (6): 52–54.

———. 1997. The ocular effects of ultraviolet radiation. *Sports Vision* 12 (3): 15–31.

Elmurr, P., Cornell, E., and Heard, R. 1996. Quantitative analyses of horizontal saccadic eye movement: Reaction times of table tennis players and non-players. *International Journal of Sports Vision* 3 (1): 46–53.

Farnsworth, C. 1997. *See it and sink it: Mastering putting through peak visual performance.* New York: Harper Collins.

Fogt, N., Uhlig, R., Thack, D.P, and Liu, A. 2002. The influence of head movement on the accuracy of a rapid pointing task. *Optometry* 73 (11): 665–673.

Giovanazzi, G. 1995. Seeing is believing: Vision is the key element to nearly all facets of the game. *Volleyball* 6 (11): 78–100.

Godnig, E.C. 2001. Body alarm reaction and sports vision. *Journal of Behavioral Optometry* 12:3–6.

Gregg, J. 1987. *Vision and sports: An introduction.* Philadelphia: Butterworth.

Hall, C., Moore, J., Annett, J., and Rodgers, W. 1997. Recalling demonstrated and guided movements using imaginary and verbal rehearsal strategies. *Research Quarterly for Exercise and Sport* 68 (2): 136–144.

Hazel, C.A. 1995. The efficacy of sports vision practice and its role in clinical optometry. *Clinical Experimental Optometry* 78:98–105.

Kopp, J.D. 1999. Eye on the ball: An interview with Dr. C. Stephen Johnson and Mark McGwire. *Journal of the American Optometric Association* 70 (2): 79–84.

Kunicki, M., and Elmurr, P. 2000. Can eye–hand coordination be trained using the AcuVision 1000? In *Proceedings of the 2000 Pre-Olympic Congress on Sports Medicine and Physical Education and International Congress on Sport Science.* Brisbane, Australia: Australian Sports Commission.

Lampert, L. 1998. *The pro's edge: Vision training for golf.* Boca Raton, FL: Saturn Press.

Martin, W. 1993. *An insight to sports.* Seattle: Sports Vision.

Montes, M.M., Bueno, I., Candel, J., and Pons, A.M. 2000. Eye–hand and eye–foot visual reaction times of young soccer players. *Optometry* 71 (12): 775–780.

Nason, P.J. 1997. M"eye" view on baseball bat speed. *Sports Vision* 13 (2): 45–47.

Press, L.J. 1997. *Applied concepts in vision therapy.* St. Louis: Mosby.

Revien, L., and Gabor, M. 1981. *Sportsvision.* New York: Workman.

Roetert, P. 1997. Keeping your eye on the ball. *Sports Vision* 13 (3): 22–23.

Schwartz, C.A. 1994. Sports screening for success. *Optometric Economics* 4 (5): 12–15.

Seiderman, A., and Schneider, S. 1983. *The athletic eye: Improved sports performance through visual training.* New York: Hearst Books.

Sherman, A. 1990. Sports vision testing and enhancement: Implications for winter sports. In *Winter sports medicine,* edited by M. Casey, C. Foster, and E. Hixson, pp. 78–84. Philadelphia: F.A. Davis.

Stahl, J. 2001. Eye–head coordination and the variation of eye-movement accuracy with orbital eccentricity. *Experimental Brain Research* 136:200–210.

Vinger, P.F. 1998. Sports medicine and the eye care professional. *Journal of the American Optometric Association* 69 (6): 395–413.

Watts, R.G., and Bahill, A.T. 2000. *Keep your eye on the ball: Curveballs, knuckleballs and fallacies of baseball.* New York: Freeman.

Wilson, T.A. 1997. Sports vision: Getting into the game. *Optometric Management Supplement* 32 (4): 20–22.

Wood, J.M., and Abernathy, B. 1997. An assessment of the efficacy of sports vision training programs. *Optometric Visual Science* 74 (8): 646–659.

INDEX

ABOUT THE AUTHORS

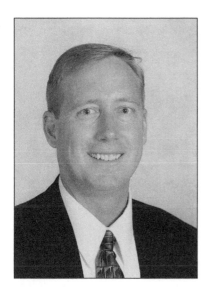

Thomas A. Wilson, OD, FCOVD, is an optometrist in Colorado Springs, Colorado. A fellow of the College of Optometrists in Vision Development, he has successfully completed an extensive postgraduate curriculum and is certified with a specialty in binocular vision. He has served as a sports vision consultant with the United States Air Force Academy, USA Shooting, and the University of Colorado ski team.

Dr. Wilson is a member of the Sports Vision section of the American Optometric Association and a former board member and exam board member for the College of Optometrists in Vision Development. He earned a FCOVD in binocular vision in 1991. In 1987, he was named Outstanding Clinician by Pacific University.

Jeff Falkel, PhD, PT, CSCS, *D, is a certified strength and conditioning specialist, exercise specialist, and sports medicine professional. Currently he serves as a physical therapist and exercise physiologist with VDP Enterprises in Littleton, Colorado. He has been a sports vision consultant for youth, high school, college, and professional athletes.

Dr. Falkel earned a PhD in exercise physiology from the University of Pittsburgh. He is an ACSM-certified exercise specialist. He was awarded the Certified Strength and Conditioning Specialist with Distinction (CSCS, *D) credential by the National Strength and Conditioning Association.

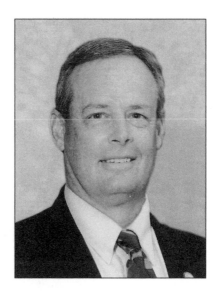

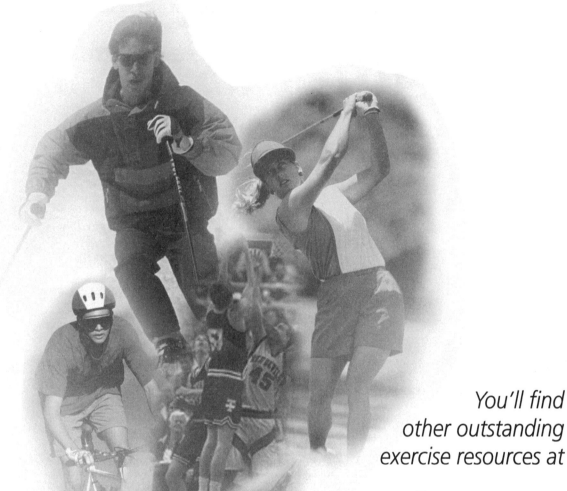